HEALTH GUIDE
for the
NUCLEAR AGE

Peter Bunyard

PAPERMAC

to my children
Paul, Maria Luisa, Amyra and Zohar
as well as to my wife
Nedira

Copyright © 1988 Roxby General Books Limited
Text Copyright © 1988 Peter Bunyard

Created by Roxby General Books Limited
a division of Roxby Press Limited
126 Victoria Rise
London SW4 0NW

Editor: John Clark
Design: Eric Drewery
Typesetting: MFK Typesetting Limited
Origination: Belmont Press
Printed by Mladinska Knjiga, Ljubljana, Yugoslavia

First published 1988 by
PAPERMAC
a division of Macmillan Publishers Limited
4 Little Essex Street London WC2R 3LF
and Basingstoke

Associated companies in Auckland, Delhi, Dublin, Gaborone,
Hamburg, Harare, Hong Kong, Johannesburg, Kuala Lumpur,
Lagos, Manzini, Melbourne, Mexico City, Nairobi, New York,
Singapore and Tokyo

British Library Cataloguing-in-Publication Data
Bunyard, Peter
Health guide for the nuclear age
I. Organisma. Effects of radiation
I. Title
574.19'15

ISBN 0–333–47305–1

HEALTH GUIDE
for the
NUCLEAR AGE

Contents

Foreword

Scientists responsible for the development of nuclear power have often insisted that, of all pollutants, radioactivity is the best understood and the least likely to cause any unexpected problems. Yet following the accident at Chernobyl there were some scientists who forecast that the eventual number of cancers caused by the fall-out would be in the region of a million, whereas others were prepared to put the figure at less than ten thousand. There was even greater uncertainty about effects of the radiation on human embryos and germ cells, and nobody seemed to know how long certain components of the environment would remain radioactive. In short, nobody seemed to know how many persons would eventually be affected, or when levels of radiation in soil, plants and animals would revert to normal.

Research carried out thirty years ago by a research department of Oxford University showed that a single X-ray taken shortly before birth was sufficient to increase the risk of an early cancer death. This finding was tantamount to discovering that there was no such thing as a safe exposure to ionizing radiation. But for nuclear scientists to have admitted this would have meant altering their perception of nuclear fission as a safe (as well as cheap) source of energy.

Even after confirmation of the Oxford finding by other scientists, several years elapsed before any official notice was taken, and we are still witnessing similar attempts to belittle any research which suggests that human tissues are more sensitive to cancer effects of radiation than The International Commission on Radiological Protection is prepared to admit. Meanwhile the fact that embryonic tissues are exceptionally vulnerable (which nobody denies) means that whenever there is substantial leakage of radioactivity from nuclear installations there will necessarily be some extra deaths masquerading as naturally-occurring birth defects or childhood cancers.

With some justification members of the public are becoming increasingly concerned about leukaemia clusters in the vicinity of some nuclear installations, and are beginning to express doubts about the reassurances coming from official sources. These reactions are signs of increasing awareness that we are now facing not only the prospect of more Chernobyls, but also the prospect of mounting levels of background radiation from *permitted* releases of radioactivity from an ever-increasing number of power plants.

In his exceptionally well illustrated book Peter Bunyard tells us, in easily understood terms, the important facts about radiation and health.

Therefore we can both arm ourselves with knowledge about what to do should we again find ourselves in the path of a radioactive plume, and also begin to understand why it is not possible to estimate the full cost of making the world increasingly dependent upon nuclear power.

Alice Stewart

Alice Stewart, MD. FRCP
Senior Research Fellow
Birmingham University

AUTHOR'S ACKNOWLEDGEMENTS

I am grateful to Grazyna Cooper and Nicholas Hildyard for their invaluable help in the preparation of this book, and to Eleanor O'Hanlow for providing excellent German translations, as well as to all at Roxby and Eric Drewery for their sustained enthusiasm and ideas. Also to Jill Raphaeline, Olivia Thomas and Ray Burrows for the illustrations.

How to use this book

A major problem in the immediate aftermath of the Chernobyl disaster was the inadequacy of monitoring facilities and the lack of information in many parts of Europe, both East and West. Many people were put unnecessarily at risk because of the poor preparation on the part of the authorities in the various countries, and in some instances by the deliberate withholding of information.

Yet much of that exposure could have been avoided if those at risk had been properly warned and advised what to do. The purpose of this book is to give practical advice, so that people can take the initiative and protect themselves and their families. What we need to know is how much fall-out has there been and where has it landed. What about the outside air, is that contaminated? Is there any risk inside buildings? What foods are safe to eat? Should we eat only garden produce, or canned food? What about imported food – can we trust it? These and many other questions are bound to trouble us after a nuclear accident involving a major escape of radiation. And Chernobyl has taught us a few lessons.

But before reacting to such a situation, we need to know something about radioactivity and where it comes from. We also need to know about the effects of radioactivity on the human body. This handbook first deals with the essential difference between natural radioactivity (to which we are all subjected) and radioactivity that has escaped from man-made installations such as nuclear reactors and nuclear reprocessing plants. Then it gives an account of the various kinds of nuclear installations and how they might go wrong. Maps show the location and type of the main installations, so that the reader can better assess the risks following an accident in a particular nuclear plant. Finally the book deals with radioactive contamination of the environment, and offers practical advice about what to do should action be necessary. Information is given about likely contamination levels in various foodstuffs following an accident and radioactive fall-out, so that the reader can make a quick and easy assessment of the risks and decide what action to take, if necessary.

Introduction

Everyone lives in a radioactive world. Indeed there would be no life at all if it were not for the atomic transformations that have taken place in the Universe since it came into being some 15 thousand million years ago. All kinds of radiations are products of these transformations. The Big Bang, the first explosive moments of our Universe, created the entire range of different atoms – from tiny hydrogen to the much more massive uranium – that later came together in forming the stars and planets, including the Earth.

Many atoms are stable, remaining intact through all the physical and chemical processes they take part in. Others, however, are inherently unstable and spontaneously transform into a new state by ejecting particles and energy from their atomic nuclei. This process, first discovered in the nineteenth century, is now known as radioactivity. Not only is radioactivity a natural phenomenon, in certain respects it is essential to the continued existence of much of life on Earth. Earthquakes, volcanoes, the thrusting up of mountains, the shifting of continents through tectonic plate movements are all powered by the enormous sum of energies from the natural disintegration of atoms such as uranium in the Earth's core. If it were not for that restless activity in the Earth deep beneath our feet, life on land may well have ground to a halt as essential nutrients were leached out of the soil and washed away into the oceans.

But there is a price to pay for the life-enhancing, beneficial effects of radioactive transformations. Radiation from a disintegrating atom can cause havoc if it strikes cells in the body, leaving a stream of chemical changes in its wake. Very often the chemical damage to a cell is sufficient to kill it. And even if the cell survives the initial trauma of radiation, it may become deranged in some way so that in time it forms a mass of cancerous tissue. In effect, cancers, genetic malformations, premature aging and early death are all potential consequences of being exposed to radiation. Yet we, as living creatures, have had no choice but to accept certain levels of radiation as an inevitable part of our environment, and to adapt to it as best as possible.

Fortunately, we are shielded from the worse effects of natural radiation. A layer of ozone high in the atmosphere filters out one type of radiation – ultraviolet light from the Sun – and prevents much of it from reaching the Earth's surface. And the soil and rocks under our feet act as a barrier to the radiation emitted by naturally occurring substances in the Earth's crust, such as uranium, radium and radon.

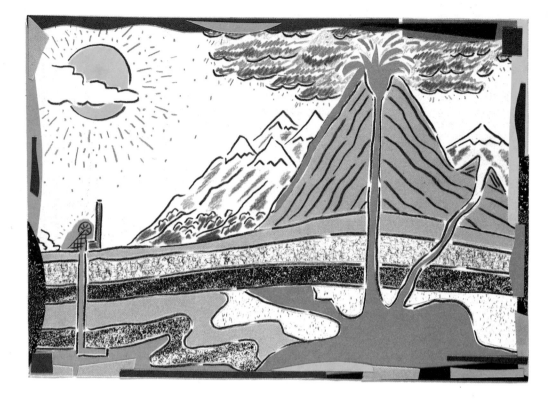

Even with all that shielding and protection, every one of us is subjected to a staggering amount of radiation in our normal lives. From a combination of cosmic radiation and naturally occuring radioactive substances in food, air, water, soil and building materials, we receive on average some 60,000 radiation strikes every second. Some of this is sufficiently energetic to pass right through us, whereas other forms get stopped dead in their tracks somewhere in the body. Over the course of a year, such natural radiation totals two thousand million events.

Obviously, if the human body did not possess a means of repairing such an onslaught of damaging rays and particles, we would not survive for long. In general cells killed by radiation are replaced by new ones resulting from normal cell division, while others that remain alive are patched up and made good. The problem is that our bodies do not always get the repair absolutely right, and the cell may become malignant and grow in an uncontrolled way, over time giving rise to a tumorous mass. On the other hand, a radiation-damaged sex cell – a sperm or ovum – may give rise to a birth defect in the offspring or result in the death of the foetus.

Modern medicine, with its use of X-rays, may now be second to natural background sources as the origin of radiation in the world. But today we are also increasingly exposed to abnormal levels of radiation resulting from scientific advances that have taken place through deliberate splitting of the atom. For instance, the atmospheric testing of hundreds of nuclear bombs during the 1950s and 1960s sprinkled the Earth with a fine dust of radioactive particles. Nuclear power stations are a mainly peaceful application of

Radioactivity is a natural part of life. The Sun's heat and light are derived from atomic transformations as is the heat that causes volcanic eruptions and the restless movement of the Earth's crust. Mountains and volcanoes replenish the land with minerals, some of which we seek in our mines. But there is a price to pay for natural radiation – in congenital malformation and disease.

splitting the atom. Such plants have routine emissions of radioactive substances as well as occasional accidental ones, the worst to date being from the Chernobyl disaster of April 1986.

Inevitably such releases will add to the toll of radiation-induced disease affecting the human population. While nuclear power stations continue to operate in the world, some within a few kilometres of where people live, we must be aware that a catastrophic accident may leave us suddenly exposed to a high level of radiation. Not only will the air be radioactive, but so will the soil, water and food. Ultimately, for the assured health of our children and their children, we may prefer to do away with nuclear power. But the right decisions must depend on knowledge and awareness. Hopefully this book will prove useful in achieving both those goals while providing a basis for action and survival.

CHAPTER

~1~

What is radiation?

Every moment of our lives we are subjected to radiation of many kinds. The different effects that this continual bombardment has on the body depends on a variety of factors, including the length of exposure and, of course, the type of radiation involved. Ultraviolet radiation from the Sun's rays, for instance, is relatively easy to guard against – suntan lotion and shade offer necessary protection. This sort of radiation is known as non-ionizing radiation, because it does not normally cause fundamental changes to atomic structure.

In this book we are concerned primarily with the class of radiation called ionizing radiation, which alters the atomic structure of substances it encounters as it travels – often at the speed of light – away from the radiation source. This kind of radiation is also known as radioactivity because of its association with the spontaneous change of one kind of atom into another, accompanied by the release of particles and energy.

A normal working or domestic environment is subject to continual natural radiation events. Gamma radiation will penetrate walls, people and steel. Beta radiation will be stopped by the body. Alpha radiation, from radioactive gases seeping naturally from the ground, will be stopped by a sheet of paper and is only dangerous when taken directly into the body.

Radiation and life

Apart from cosmic radiation, which will be discussed later, alpha, beta and gamma rays are the principal forms of radiation to which people on Earth are exposed (X-rays are a less energetic form of gamma radiation).

Alpha particles are relatively heavy and ponderous, with considerable energy but little penetrating power. Despite their being blocked by no more than a sheet of paper or the outer layers of the skin, they can still cause damage at the microscopic level on account of their mass. If a gamma ray can be thought of as a high-velocity bullet, then an alpha ray is like a cannon ball. An alpha particle consists of two protons (thus giving it a double positive charge) and two neutrons. When expelled from the nucleus of an atom, it therefore carries off an effective mass of four. For instance plutonium, with a mass 239, transforms into uranium with a mass of 235 when an alpha particle is lost from its nucleus.

A beta particle, which is a high-speed electron (and therefore negatively charged), produces in human tissue an intensity of radiation that is about a thousand times less than that produced by an alpha particle. On the other hand, a beta particle travels some thousand times farther through the tissues. In terms of local radiation damage, this penetration makes up some of the difference between the two types of radiation. A piece of paper may be enough to block alpha radiation, but blocking beta requires the equivalent of a sheet of aluminium 1 millimetre thick.

Gamma rays are like powerful X-rays with extremely short wavelengths. They have high energies and penetrating powers, being able to pass through

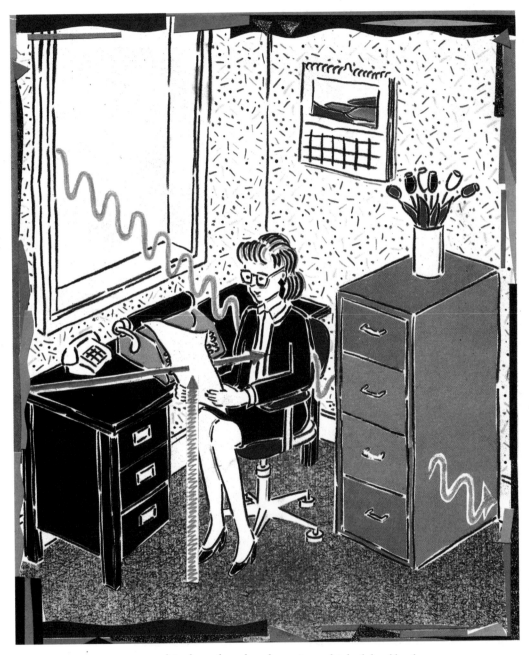

several inches of steel and require a thick slab of lead or concrete to stop them. Nuclear installations containing gamma-emitting substances need to be surrounded by a concrete containment shield. Gamma rays and X-rays are made up of particles called photons, which when they have lower energies and travel with much longer wavelengths comprise what we perceive as visible light. And being photons, gamma rays and X-rays travel at the speed of light.

Radioactive decay

If it were possible to separate out just one atom of a radioactive element, it would be impossible to predict exactly when it was likely to change into another one. Yet, when a sufficient number of unstable atoms of the element are separated out, it is possible to predict with some accuracy just how many will decay and transmute into another element.

Not surprisingly, the greater the number of the original atoms, the higher is the number that will decay in a given period of time. The time taken for half of the atoms of an isotope to decay is known as its half-life. Essentially what the half-life tells us is that it will take as long for the remaining half to decay to one quarter as it took for the original amount to decay to half.

A particular isotope has a particular half-life. Carbon-14 used in radio-carbon dating experiments has a half-life of 5,730 years. Thus one half of it decays in that amount of time, one quarter of the original quantity in another stretch of that time, one-eighth over the next period, and so on. After ten half-lives – equal to 57,300 years for carbon-14 – there will be less than one-thousandth of the original quantity left.

The half-lives of different radio-isotopes vary enormously, some being extremely short and expressed in fractions of a second, others being extended into millions of years. Barium-143 has a half-life of 12 seconds, there being only one-thousandth of the original amount left after two minutes. Iodine-129, on the other hand, has a half-life of 1.7 million years. The radioactive gas radon, which is a natural decay product of uranium-238, has a half-life of 3.82 days. Uranium-238 itself has a half-life of 4,510 million years, which means that approximately half of that present when the Earth was formed has how been transformed into other elements. In fact the radioactive decay of uranium-238 is the start of a 14-stage linked chain of transformations, finishing up with lead-206 – which is stable and therefore non-radioactive.

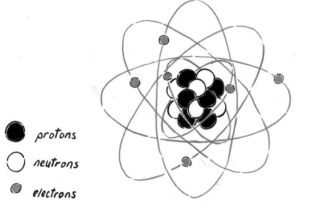

● protons

○ neutrons

◕ electrons

Atoms consist of protons and neutrons tightly bound together in the nucleus with electrons in orbit around, some close to the nucleus, others further away.

A radioactive atom decays at a consistent rate. The times it takes for half of that present to decay is known as a half-life. After 5 half-lives have gone 1/32 of the original is left.

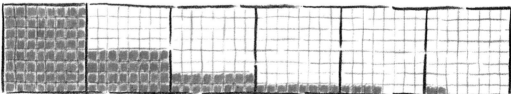

14

When a radioactive atom decays, depending on the substance concerned, different processes can take place. One involves beta decay in which an electron is expelled from the nucleus. The loss of that negatively charged beta particle/electron from the nucleus, converts a neutron into a positively charged proton. Since the number of protons determines the nature of the atom, the original atom has therefore became an atom one higher in the progressive series of atoms. Alpha radiation on the other hand, involves the expulsion of two protons or two neutrons combined together. The total mass of the original atom therefore falls by four units, while the loss of two protons takes the element two down in the atomic series. Many radioactive atoms emit gamma rays when undergoing decay and atomic transformation.

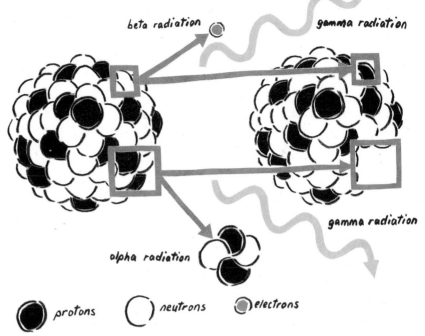

Uranium-235, the other naturally-occurring isotope of uranium, has a half-life of 700 million years. At present uranium-235 comprises no more than 0.7 per cent of uranium ore, with uranium-238 making up nearly all the rest. When the Earth was formed, there would therefore have been about a hundred times more uranium-235 than at present, and double the present amount of uranium-238, making the Earth far more radioactive then than it is now.

The radiation emitted from a radio-isotope is more intense the higher its concentration and the shorter its half-life. The kind of radiation emitted also depends on the specific radio-isotope. Carbon-14, for instance, emits beta particles to decay to nitrogen-14 (which is stable), whereas polonium-210, with a half-life of 138.4 days, emits alpha particles together with gamma rays to decay to lead-206, which is also stable.

Natural and man-made radiation

Most radioactive particles encountered in nature come from the decay products of uranium and thorium, and they include radon, thoron and polonium. All told they have long half-lives – that is, they take many years to decay into harmless substances – but very low concentrations, and as a result have a barely detectable effect on living organisms.

Meanwhile, some 1,000 radioactive elements have been made artificially in accelerators and nuclear reactors. Most of them tend to decay fairly rapidly, at least on a geological time-scale. But some, like niobium-94 or nickel-59, have the very long half-lives of 20,000 and 80,000 years respectively. Because they are generated in the steel used to construct reactors, they add to the problems of dismantling the installation at the end of its life and disposing of the pieces.

A nuclear reactor operates through the splitting of certain atoms, which are known as fissile because of the relative ease with which they fragment when struck by a neutron. The most widely used fissile materials are uranium-235 and plutonium-239, which itself first has to be generated in another nuclear reactor. When splitting into fragments, such fissile atoms also shed several neutrons – which can then be used to keep the nuclear chain reaction going. The fragments are themselves radioactive elements which emit alpha, beta and gamma radiation as well as neutrons.

ᛵᛵᛵ How does radiation affect us? ᛵᛵᛵ

Although we are able to detect the shape and physical structure – if not the taste – of substances that are radioactive, we cannot sense the radiation they emit. We can therefore hold a piece of radium or uranium in our hand without knowing that it is radioactive. And even if some of the radiation emitted is in the visible light range, like the yellow glow from uranium salts, it is insufficient to make us blink or shut our eyes. Indeed, in our normal, daily existence we are not usually subjected to high levels of ionizing radiation from radioactive substances and therefore our bodies have never needed to develop radiation detectors that will enable us to take avoiding action.

In 1987 some members of a family in Brazil died as a result of becoming heavily irradiated with gamma rays after a scrap dealer opened an abandoned capsule containing a radiation source for a hospital cancer therapy machine. There was nothing to warn them that they were exposing themselves to lethal doses of radiation.

If we are subjected to a high enough dose of radiation over a relatively short space of time, such as over the course of a few minutes or a day, we are likely to become sick within a few hours and we may die, sometimes after a prolonged illness. The effects of high radiation doses – such as severe headaches, diarrhoea, reddening and blistering of the skin, followed by hair falling out and even unconsciousness – are tangible signs of irradiation that leave little doubt as to the cause.

On the other hand the effects of low doses of radiation are exceedingly difficult to follow, especially as they may take years to manifest themselves. Cancer is one consequence of having been subjected to radiation; genetic effects leading to congenital malformations in offspring or to the death of a foetus may be another. But how can one distinguish between a cancer or genetic defect caused by exposure to ionizing radiation and ones brought on by other environmental causes such as exposure to toxic chemicals?

Radiation and cancer
Laboratory experiments on animals indicate that exposure to radiation usually causes cancer at a particular rate, but the question then arises as to whether the animals used are sufficiently comparable in their response to radiation for the results to be valid in human beings – especially because the doses used tend to be high. The unravelling of the likely number of cancers caused in human populations by ionizing radiation is fraught with problems because no one person or group is exactly comparable to another. Neverthe-

16

In today's world, in which we are subjected to many different cancer producing substances, it is very difficult to isolate any one as being the actual cause of cancer in the individual.

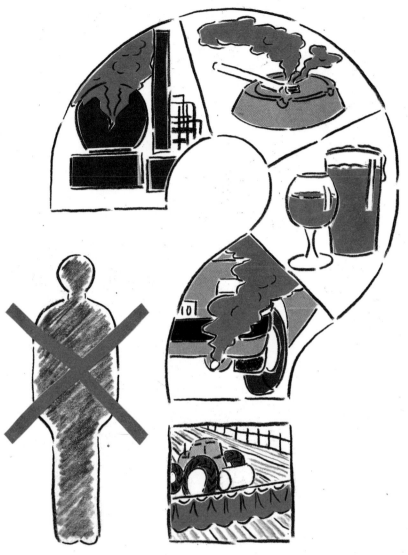

less, such studies are part and parcel of the science of epidemiology, in which human populations are studied for their medical history, and as more and more experience accumulates the indications are that there really is a link between exposure to even low doses of radiation and a raised incidence of cancer (as well as of congenital defects).

Ionizing radiation

What are the effects of ionizing radiation? The substantial difference between ionizing and non-ionizing radiation is that only ionizing radiation has sufficient energy to strip electrons away from their positions around an atomic nucleus. Once an electron has been blasted away, the chemical characteristics of the atom are radically altered and it can engage in new interactions.

Some small chemical compounds such as water turn into highly reactive substances called free radicals after being ionized. The free radicals then very quickly interact with other chemical compounds in their vicinity. In a living cell, where structure and organization are of paramount importance in the maintenance of normal activities, any change is likely to be detrimental. Depending on the part of the cell affected, ionizing radiation can be lethal, and destroy biochemical processes upon which the cell relies.

Being electrically charged, both alpha and beta particles have a direct effect in causing ionization. Neutrons, which have no charge, cause ionization by knocking out protons. Because hydrogen is composed essentially of protons, it is a likely target for neutrons, the hydrogen losing its electron and becoming a proton with almost as much energy as the original neutron. The electron-less hydrogen atom can therefore cause ionization in a similar way to alpha particles with their double protons. Some neutrons may get captured by atoms, destabilizing them so that they emit alpha or beta radiation with a gamma ray. Finally the photons in gamma or cosmic rays have sufficient energies along their trajectories to knock out electrons and cause ionization.

The amount of ionization caused by a single X-ray is truly astonishing. Today, with the best X-ray machines, doses have been reduced to a tenth or even a twentieth of what they were before the 1960s, when a chest X-ray could involve a dose of as much as one rad (a rad is defined as the amount of radiation that will deliver 100 ergs of energy per gram of matter). One rad of X-rays would produce as many as two million ionization events in human tissues. Rads are no longer used as the unit of dose, having been replaced by the gray, which is equivalent to 100 rads.

Radiation damage to the body

Not unexpectedly, the large number of ionizations from an X-ray causes damage. One place to look for this is at the lymphocytes (types of white blood cells), which can be drawn off in a drop of blood and cultured outside the body. Indeed one millilitre of human blood contains more than a million of such white cells, and by special tissue culture techniques scientists can observe the nuclei of the cells and their chromosomes, and check whether they are damaged.

Chromosomes carry the cell's genes, which are responsible for organizing the cell's activities and for defining what kind of cell it is – whether a blood cell, liver cell, lung cell, gut cell, or whatever. The chromosomes and the genetic material they bear in the form of DNA (deoxyribonucleic acid) have been found to be particularly vulnerable to ionization caused by radiation. For instance, the ionization of water molecules, which are major components of all living cells, leads to the formation of free oxygen, hydrogen peroxide and extremely active substances such as hydroxyl. All of these interact very rapidly with the chromosomes, causing breakages with the resulting loss of bits of chromosomal material or the wrong pieces becoming attached to each other.

Such changes have been detected in human lymphocytes that have been irradiated after being taken from the body. They have also been found in the blood of human beings who either by accident or as a result of routine exposure to radioactive substances have received measurable radiation.

Not that radiation is the only cause of such abnormalities. They can

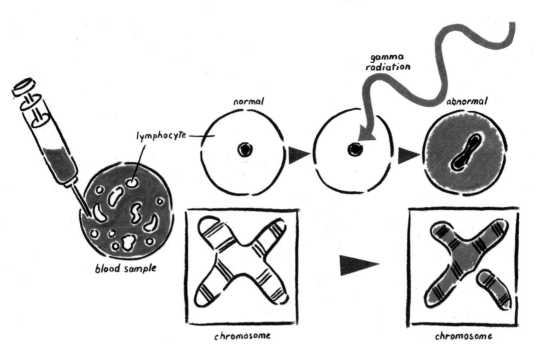

lymphocyte

blood sample

gamma radiation

normal

abnormal

chromosome

chromosome

result from exposure to many different kinds of pollutants, including cigarette smoke and diesel fumes. Therefore before we can estimate what ionizing radiation does to the cells – and in particular to the chromosomes – we have to know how much damage if any is to be found in normal unexposed people. In fact, if we examine the chromosomes of lymphocyte cells taken from young adults who do not smoke but of course are exposed to traffic fumes and other industrial pollutants, we find that approximately one per cent of the cells have damaged chromosomes involving breakages, losses and rearrangements. As we age, the proportion of cells showing such damage increases, and may be as high as 5 or 6 per cent in 60-year-olds.

When lymphocytes are taken from the body and subjected to X-rays, they appear to withstand radiation doses of up to 5 rads without showing any detectable increase in the proportion damaged. At higher X-ray doses, damage begins to show up, with marked increases up to about 35 rads and then a fall-off in the rate of increase as the radiation dose gets to 50 rads.

On the other hand, studies of the chromosomes in white blood cells taken from men working in naval dockyards where nuclear submarines are repaired indicate that, even though the men are exposed to levels of radiation well within the occupational limit of 5 rads per year, the number of detectable chromosomal aberrations goes up significantly. This is unlike the study with X-rays, which indicated that a threshold is in operation up to doses of 5 rads. Not that such changes are unique to radiation damage. Similar studies on cigarette smokers demonstrate that the damage to chromosomes from inhaling the smoke is equivalent to being exposed to 1 to 2 rads of ionizing radiation per year.

For the most part, the naval dockers are exposed to gamma rays, which have considerably higher energies than X-rays. Normal people may be able to repair much of the damage to their cells when the radiation dose is low and when the energies are in the range associated with X-rays. Such repair may get increasingly difficult as the energies increase and particularly when particles such as alpha and beta are involved. An increased rate of cancer is one of the consequences of being exposed to radiation, but doctors do not yet know precisely the course of events that leads up to the disease.

One suggestion is that the cells fail to repair properly damage to the chromosomes, and so normal control of the cell's activities is lost. Through continuing cell division, a colony of aberrant cells is formed which, over time, forms a malignant mass that invades and destroys healthy tissues.

Another suggestion is that the impact of radiation on the chromosomes enables certain genes – which until then had been dormant – to become active and express themselves. These genes, known as oncogenes, then unleash the processes of aberrant cell division that underlie cell cancer. Viruses similar to oncogenes have also been implicated, and it may well turn out that a number of different processes are involved in the formation of cancers, some operating alone, some together.

How sensitive are we to radiation?

How radiation affects us depends on the type and intensity of the radiation, and whether our whole body or just part of it has been exposed. Basically, ionizing radiation is divided into two broad categories. One type has a relatively high penetrating power, but leaves a sparse amount of ionization at any one point along its path through tissues. And the other has little penetrating power, but its impact on the tissues produces a great many ionizations before it loses its energy.

A problem in trying to find the link between radiation exposure and cancer is the long delay – sometimes several decades – before the cancer is noticed, by which time it may prove difficult to treat. In fact, for the first few years after the Hiroshima and Nagasaki atomic bombs were dropped on Japan, the numbers of additional cancers (above the normal rate) among the survivors was barely detectable. Indeed, members of the Atomic Bomb Casualty Commission, who had been sent from the United States to investigate the residual effects of the bombs, came to the conclusion in the mid-1950s that, apart from a few extra cases of leukaemia, the surviving populations of the two cities were back to normal with regards to health.

For the United States and the other superpowers, at that time developing their nuclear arsenals, such a find was reassuring. It seemed to suggest that, given adequate shelter from the blast, the human population might survive a limited nuclear war. However, Dr Alice Stewart of the Cancer Registry at Birmingham University points out the pitfall of using the Hiroshima and Nagasaki data as if the surviving population was normal and comparable in all respects with other populations in Japan and the rest of the world. In fact the survivors of these bombs were exceptional. Not only had they survived the initial blast and high levels of radiation when hundreds of thousands of others had succumbed, but they had also continued to survive through a winter in devastated cities with poor nutrition and the most meagre of medical care. Moreover, that was in the days before antibiotics were in common use. Alice Stewart has called such people 'healthy survivors', because they must have been exceptionally fit before the blast, and their hardiness enabled them to survive against all odds.

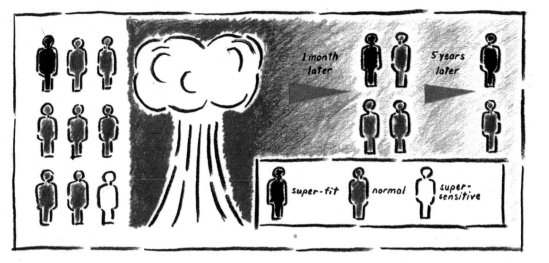

super-fit *normal* *super-sensitive*

Some people are much better able to stand large doses of radiation. Others are extremely sensitive. As a result the population of survivors from the Hiroshima and Nagasaki bombs tended to include a higher proportion of 'super-fit people' among them. Any study of radiation on the human population must therefore take the 'healthy survivor effect' into account.

Nevertheless the Hiroshima and Nagasaki survivors represented the largest population by far to have been subjected to acute radiation. Scientists with the Atomic Bomb Casualty Commission clearly found it tempting to use the data they had collected for drawing general conclusions concerning the relationship between exposure to radiation and the additional cancers that would result. In fact the Commission began its study only in 1950, five years after the bombs had been dropped, during which time many people, with somewhat less resilience than the healthy survivors, had died.

Short-term effects

One effect of radiation may be to impair the body's immune system so that not only cancers but also other diseases – in particular infectious diseases – can develop and become fatal. AIDS – the auto-immune deficiency syndrome that is caused by the human immunodeficiency virus (HIV) – has just such an effect and its victims are likely to develop cancers and serious infectious diseases simultaneously. Death in the end is likely to result from infection rather than from cancer.

Alice Stewart and others have surmised that many of those who survived the atomic bomb blast but died between 1945 and 1950 (in the period before the Atomic Bomb Casualty Commission began its study) may have been already developing cancer but became excessively vulnerable to infection before the cancer could manifest itself. For the victims and their families, the final cause of death is not likely to be the most important factor. For an epidemiologist who studies disease patterns in populations and tries to elucidate why they occur, the cause of death is highly relevant.

In effect, any conclusions drawn from the Hiroshima and Nagasaki data concerning the effect of acute doses of radiation on health and the length of life are likely to be optimistic and underestimate the mortality from cancer and other diseases. The situation has now become even more confused following a re-evaluation of the likely radiation doses received by the survivors. Indeed, they are half as large as they were previously considered to be, therefore in one fell swoop doubling the risk from a given radiation dose. But more about risk later.

21

Tissue sensitivity

Medical experience with ionizing radiation has shown that different tissues in the body have different sensitivities regarding the risk of developing fatal cancers. Clearly the greatest risk of developing cancer results from the whole body being irradiated, because every type of tissue is affected. Radiation biologists have now come up with a risk-weighting system, which is designed to take the different tissue sensitivities into account in proportion to whole-body irradiation. For instance, if a radiation dose of 1 sievert is confined to the lung, the probability of that dose inducing a fatal cancer is considered to be approximately one-eighth that of a similar dose to the entire body. Similarly, to the thyroid, the proportional risk is considered to be one-thirtieth that of a whole-body dose. The sum of all the doses to the different tissues multiplied by a risk-weighting factor should then give what is termed the 'effective dose equivalent'.

The use of such risk-weighting factors assumes that radiation scientists have properly interpreted the data on the effects of irradiation on different

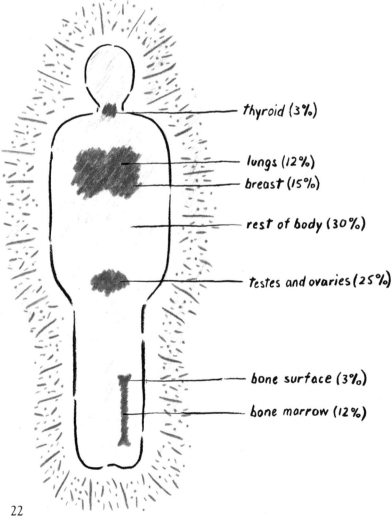

thyroid (3%)

lungs (12%)
breast (15%)

rest of body (30%)

testes and ovaries (25%)

bone surface (3%)
bone marrow (12%)

Different parts of the body have been given different ratings with regards to the risks of cancer from radiation. A dose to the thyroid is estimated to be equivalent in fatal cancer risk to 3 per cent of the same delivered over the whole body, the lung 12 per cent and so on as indicated in the diagram. The total irradiation of the body therefore adds up to 100 per cent.

groups of people. A major problem, and it applies to virtually all such data, is that the radiation doses to which humans have been exposed – whether by accident as in nuclear power incidents, whether by design as with the Hiroshima and Nagasaki victims, or whether for medical treatment as in the past use of X-rays for treating patients with the crippling bone disease ankylosing spondylitis – have always been in the high range. The assumption has then followed that the effects at low doses are directly proportional to those at high doses.

In the 1950s many radiation scientists believed that the body could cope with low doses and would efficiently carry out repairs. The notion came into being of a threshold radiation dose, below which no damage would be incurred. As pointed out earlier, our bodies do seem to cope well with low doses of low LET radiation such as X-rays and repair the damage, yet it needs no more than a few faulty repairs for an aberrant cell to break away and start growing malignantly. In effect it is the risk of those few, but not negligible, aberrations that we have to deal with in assessing the cancer risk associated with radiation. The consensus now is that we cannot assume any threshold dose, and even very low doses put us at risk from cancers and from passing on congenital malformations.

Recommended safety levels

The levels of radioactivity considered safe have come down sharply over the years. In the 1930s the authorities considered a yearly maximum dose of 75 rem acceptable. By 1987 it had been reduced 1,500 times compared with that earlier figure.

The possible harmful effects of radiation have been known for a long time. As long ago as 1896 a report in the British Medical Journal described the irritated red skin and sore eyes among early X-ray pioneers. The first victim of cumulative radiation exposure in Britain died in 1900, and during the next 30 years he was followed by more than 60 others. Meanwhile a study of leukaemia among American radiologists showed that they had a ten times greater incidence of the fatal disease than other physicians, and a similar excess was found among British radiologists. Both Madame Curie (the discover of radium) and her daughter Irene died of leukaemia caused by a long exposure to ionizing radiation.

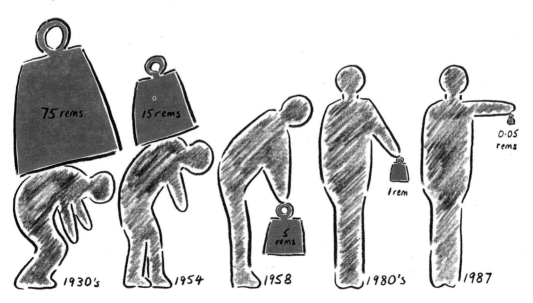

75 rems — 1930's
15 rems — 1954
5 rems — 1958
1 rem — 1980's
0.05 rems — 1987

In 1928, to put some limits on radiation exposure (particularly among physicians), the International Commission on Radiological Protection (ICRP) was established under the name International X-ray and Radium Protection Committee. After World War II and the arrival of the Atomic Age, it was not just medical staff and physicists who were becoming routinely exposed to artificial radiation, but the world at large, and the scope of the Committee had to expand into its present form.

In 1977 the ICRP introduced the notion of cost-benefit into its rationale for radiological protection. Thus it suggested that the exposure of the public to radiation from the use of nuclear power should be assessed in the light of the economic benefits derived from the use of that form of energy. It called for radiation doses to be kept 'as low as reasonably achievable, economic and social considerations being taken into account'.

Many countries, including the United States, Britain, the Soviet Union and the countries of Eastern and Western Europe, have accepted the ICRP recommendations on dose limits. But there is increasing concern among radiation scientists that these limits reflect more the nuclear industry's need to be able to operate economically than the need to give full protection to the public. Obviously any assessment of cost-benefit depends essentially on the estimate of risk to health from radiation, and what if the ICRP has got such risk assessment radically wrong, by a factor of ten or more?

Over the past 60 years the ICRP's recommended dose limits have been dramatically reduced. In 1931 the recommended maximum permissible limit for someone occupationally exposed to radiation was 75 rems a year. The limit was then successively reduced to 50 rems, then to 25; in 1954 it was reduced yet again to 15 rems and then in 1958 to 5 rems a year. It has remained at this level, but with the proviso that every effort should be made to keep exposures to workers in the nuclear industry below 0.5 rem a year. In general, maximum permissible doses to members of the public were set at one-tenth of those considered acceptable to workers in industry. Today the recommendation is that members of the public should not receive more than 1 millisievert (0.1 rem) a year from such industrial sources of radiation as nuclear power.

The cancer curve

A major point of controversy has been the precise nature of the relationship between radiation dose and the induction of cancer. Most radiation biologists agree about the cancer-causing effects of radiation when the dose is high, as in people who have received X-ray treatment for conditions such as ankylosing spondylitis or even for ringworm. But they disagree vehemently about the long-term effects on health of low doses.

The ICRP has cut through such disagreement by opting for a straightforward proportional relationship, in which each increment in radiation dose causes a proportionate increase in the likely numbers of cancers. Such a straight-line relationship has considerable advantages when calculating the likely consequences of total doses received by a given population. For instance, if 100 people receive estimated radiation doses of 1 millisievert each from an accidental release of radioactive material, then according to the straight-line relationship the total risk of cancers developing among that group would be the same as if ten people received radiation doses of 10 millisieverts each or one person received a dose of 100 millisieverts. Since

Scientists still do not know how many people are likely to develop cancer as a result of low dose radiation. The model used by the authorities, suggests that the numbers affected will be strictly proportional to the dose. On the other hand the evidence increasingly suggests that as indicated in the lower group four or even ten times more may be affected by low radiation doses.

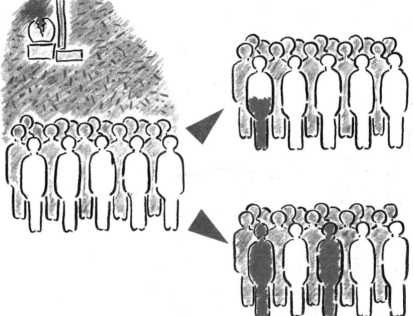

statistics are involved, any relationship between dose and its effects is likely to hold better when the population under study is large.

In fact, because the ICRP and public bodies such as Britain's National Radiological Protection Board employ the straight-line relationship, they can readily calculate what is termed the collective effective dose equivalent and then make estimates of the numbers of cancers likely to accrue in the population concerned. Indeed the collective effective dose equivalent can be derived from totting up the radiation dose after it has been adjusted by both radiation quality factors and risk-weighting factors to all members of an exposed population. The risk of cancer among that population depends on the collective total. From the point of view of the researcher rather than the exposed person, it does not change even if one person receives ten or more times as much radiation as another person.

But what if the relationship is not a straightforward one, and instead lower doses of radiation are ten or twenty times more effective in causing cancers per unit of radiation than are higher doses? If that situation prevails, the use of collective effective dose equivalents gives an entirely misleading estimate of the collective cancer risk. In that respect, 100 people receiving 1 millisievert each have a much greater risk of developing cancer than ten people receiving ten times the dose, even though the collective effective dose is the same in both cases.

Such a discussion is by no means academic, because there is increasing evidence data that small radiation doses are significantly more effective in inducing cancers than are larger ones. And if that evidence is widely accepted as more representative of reality, the estimates of the numbers of people throughout Scandinavia and Europe who are likely to suffer premature death as a result of the radioactive fall-out from Chernobyl will have to be increased by a factor of ten or more.

Radiation and its effects on pregnancy and children

Of all people, an unborn child is the most vulnerable to radiation. There is evidence that a foetus is at least ten times more sensitive to radiation in terms of the incidence of cancer than the general population. Sensitivity is probably highest in the first three months of pregnancy, when the various foetal tissues are forming. For this reason, any woman who is pregnant should take extra care to avoid unnecessary exposure to radiation – for example, to X-rays or to cosmic rays at high altitudes (as in a high-flying aircraft).

The first indication of how sensitive a foetus is came from the pioneering work of Dr Alice Stewart, which was derided at first but is now accepted as proving a link between radiation and childhood cancer. In 1955, as a researcher in social medicine, Alice Stewart set out to determine why the incidence of leukaemia in children had increased significantly at the end of World War II. Was it because of better diagnosis? Or was it perhaps that better forms of treatment kept children alive who previously would have died from some other cause before their leukaemia was diagnosed? She was particularly interested in the role that antibiotics would have played in changing the pattern of disease in the general population.

The chief culprit turned out to be X-rays administered to women in early pregnancy. Stewart discovered that a single X-ray dose of some 0.25 rads (2.5 milligrays) given to mothers-to-be had caused a 25 per cent increase in the later development of childhood leukaemias and cancers. Before the war and the general use of antibiotics, children with a pre-cancerous condition – and therefore with a weakened immune system – succumbed to infections such as respiratory disorders. After the war, antibiotics successfully treated such disorders until the cancer manifested itself. On Dr Stewart's figures, if all pregnant women were subjected to half a millisievert of ionizing radiation in addition to natural background radiation, there would be an additional 20 per cent or more of childhood cancers, equivalent to an extra 130 cases for every million live births.

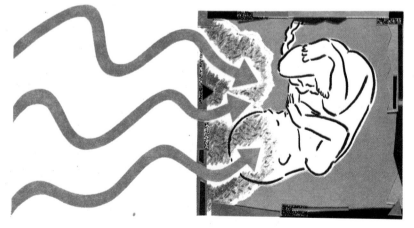

The developing child in the womb is particularly vulnerable to ionizing radiation such as X-rays.

~~~~ Children at risk ~~~~

Dr Stewart's conclusions may explain why the childhood cancer rate has been very much higher than expected in regions where there have been discharges of radioactive materials. But the effects of radiation on pregnant women are not limited merely to cancer and the the extra vulnerability of infants to disease. Inherited disorders and congenital malformations are another problem.

Inherited disorders are those that we, usually unwittingly, pass on to our children. Characteristics – good and bad – are inherited through the genes, which are basically strands of chemicals that act as a code for controlling the actions of cells within the body. Genes can be affected by small, inconspicuous alterations to their structure, and such structural changes can be induced by ionizing radiation. Genes are carried on chromosomes, and these in turn are located in the nuclei of cells. If the disordered cell is a sex cell (the egg of a woman or the sperm of a man), genetic and chromosomal abnormalities can arise in the offspring.

For instance, a gross visible change to a chromosome occurs in Down's syndrome (also called mongolism or trisomy 21), in which one chromosome has an extra piece attached to it. Chromosomal mutations may be responsible for as many as one out of every two spontaneous miscarriages in early pregnancy, and for a small percentage of congenital abnormalities among live births. Small-point mutations probably cause most hereditary disorders, which are known to affect at least ten per cent of all live births.

The United Nations Scientific Committee on the Effects of Atomic Radiation (UNSCEAR) consider the risk for hereditary damage to human beings to be two from every 100 sieverts of radiation dose delivered to a population. It is assumed to apply to future generations. Not all people will have children after being irradiated, and so the risk of serious hereditary defects over the first two generations reduces to one-fifth of the overall risk factor – that is, to 1 in 250 per sievert.

Certain tissues are more sensitive to radiation than others. So the health risk following irradiation of the gonads (in which sex cells are formed) is given a weighting factor – primarily to take account of the potential hereditary harm that might result. For this reason UNSCEAR estimates that the overall whole-body risk, including both cancer and hereditary effects, is 1 in 60 per sievert, or 165 for every 10,000 person sieverts dose to the population.

If an embryo inherits gross genetic faults from one or both of its parents, it is likely to miscarry. But some affected foetuses go to full term and are stillborn or born with congenital malformations. If men and women are subjected to a radiation dose of only half a millisievert per year from a nuclear installation – the maximum level now being called for by some regulatory bodies – the result is likely to be an increase in heriditary effects of 1 or 2 per cent. Pre-World War II radiologists, who took fewer precautions in protecting themselves from X-rays and were exposed to several hundred millisieverts each year, parented children with a higher incidence of malformations.

It is therefore obvious that children are those who are most at risk from radiation. Indeed the debility and sickness resulting from congenital disease

27

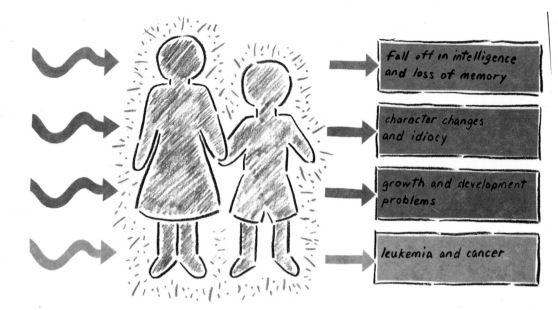

	Fall off in intelligence and loss of memory
	character changes and idiocy
	growth and development problems
	leukemia and cancer

or cancer derived from irradiation of the foetus in the womb occur when we are children, because with such disorders the chances of a full life as an adult are much reduced. The actual additional numbers involved may be no more than a few per cent of all live births, but this in no way diminishes their significance.

As well as cancer and congenital malformations, ionizing radiation can cause other developmental problems in children. Growth, for instance, can be halted or lead to deformity when cartilage or bone is irradiated, although the amount of radiation needs to be in the order of several grays over an extended period.

Mental retardation and a reduction in the diameter of the baby's head can also follow an acute radiation dose during development in the womb. Such defects were found among one-quarter of all children born to Japanese bomb survivors pregnant at the time of the explosions.

There is also evidence that children subjected to high radiation doses to the skull show a number of mental changes, including a fall-off in intelligence, loss of memory, character changes and in the very young dementia and idiocy. One study of children who received both drugs and cranial X-rays to treat acute lymphocytic leukaemia revealed a sudden, sharp decline in intelligence quotient (IQ) some 2 years after the diagnosis of the disease. The decline was greatest in children who were under 5 years old when treated. Another group of children who received only drug treatment (and no X-rays) maintained their IQ throughout. The implication therefore is that the X-rays – admittedly in the high range of 24 grays overall – were responsible for affecting mental ability.

Controversy about the effects of radiation on the body, particularly the genetic and cancer effects, will undoubtedly remain. Yet the evidence, however circumstantial, continues to build up. Thus in April 1987 the Human Genetics Institute of West Berlin published its findings for 1986 on

As the radiation dose increases so the level of damage to the child consequently rises.

a nationwide survey of genetic malformations in the foetus. The survey was made on samples obtained by amniocentesis, a technique in which cells from the amniotic fluid surrounding the foetus are studied using a microscope. It showed that the highest incidence for that year of Down's syndrome (trisomy-21) was in children who were conceived in early May, particularly among those parents who were in southern Germany at the time. The sudden increase in this chromosomal disorder appeared to coincide with the fall-out from the Chernobyl nuclear disaster in the Ukraine. Indeed the study was initiated after the discovery of ten babies with Down's syndrome born in West Berlin in January 1987, exactly nine months after Germany had received its sprinkling of fall-out. (Normally two Down's syndrome births would be expected.) Later enquiries revealed that of 17 babies born with the disorder in other parts of West Germany, 15 of them were from the most heavily contaminated region in the southern part of the country. All of those children were the result of conceptions that took place during the time when fall-out was at its most intense.

⏤⏤ Radiation and its effects on adults ⏤⏤

As we age, passing from a foetus inside our mother's womb through childhood, adolescence, adulthood, middle age and then old age, our susceptibility to cancer changes. Moreover, certain cancers seem to be more prominent during particular periods of our lives, and less prominent during others. In the context of this book, we can ask a number of key questions. How does exposure to ionizing radiation affect the incidence of specific cancers? Are all cancers sensitive to radiation? And does the degree of sensitivity depend on the natural incidence of the cancer concerned?

The difficulty in finding out how many cancers are caused by low doses of radiation is aggravated by what happens to us as we age. If we are exposed to excess ionizing radiation, does it merely cause a particular number of additional cancers, or does the number of extra cancers increase as we get older? The authorities assume the former. But recent data on the number of cancers among the survivors at Hiroshima and Nagasaki shows the cancer rate to be soaring, therefore implying that the rate following radiation exposure indeed does go up with age.

On the whole the relationship between cancer, radiation and the body's immune system is not clear. A healthy immune system undoubtedly serves to keep infections at bay and in all probability is an important mechanism in mopping up aberrant cancer cells. A number of scientists believe that cancer cells are being formed in our bodies throughout our lives but that they are eliminated quickly by the immune system when it recognizes them as 'foreign' cells. Such ideas are reinforced by way in which rare cancers such as Kaposi's sarcoma, a cancer of the skin, tends to be associated with AIDS and the failure of the immune system. It is probable therefore that somebody with a healthy immune system is better able to resist both infectious diseases and the constant tendency of a small number of the body's cells to form a malignant tumour. Such people may be more radiation resistant than others, and this may explain why there were survivors at Hiroshima even among those exposed to very high levels of radiation.

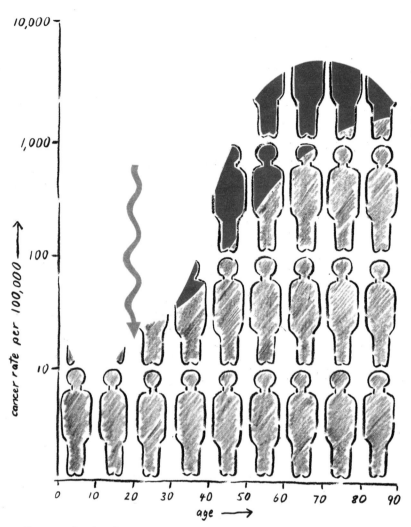

As we age the overall rate of cancer increases. As shown here, if at the age of 20 we are subjected to a radiation event, then the additional numbers of cancers are likely to follow the outline indicated in red.

Because the development of a malignant tumour appears to be strongly linked to changes in the immune system, the chances are that even before a cancer reveals its presence to the patient and doctor there will be a greater susceptibility to infectious diseases. At least such a suggestion seems to hold for children, who at the time of infection are not known to be harbouring a cancer but who later are diagnosed as having it.

Radiation as we get older
When various types of cancer are correlated with age, a definite pattern emerges in which the incidence of main cancers – such as lung cancer in men and breast cancer in women – rises from a very low level in childhood and adolescence and then peaks out in later life as other causes of death take over and become more significant. For breast cancer, there is a very rapid rise in incidence between the ages of 20 and 50, followed by a levelling off. As far as vulnerability to radiation is concerned, the risk appears to be greatest in women aged between 20 and 24, and declines after that.

30

Leukaemia is the first kind of cancer to appear after exposure to radiation, occurring within a few years at most. Some 15 years after radiation exposure, most if not all of the extra leukaemias caused by radiation seem to have manifested themselves and the leukaemia rate then returns to normal. People exposed to radiation when they are under the age of 15 develop leukaemia sooner after exposure than do those who are older (who also have a lower incidence of the disease).

⚘⚘ Workers in the nuclear industry ⚘⚘

It comes as no surprise that people employed in the nuclear industry are more likely than most of us to be exposed to above average levels of radiation. Not only are they likely to receive radiation at work, but if radioactive wastes are discharged from the nuclear plant and they live in the vicinity, they and their families also receive additional doses of radiation from that source.

Does such exposure to radiation put the workers at risk? The intention, according to the nuclear industry and radiation standard setters, is that nuclear power should be deemed a safe industry. Thus the risk of an accident or any event that shortens life should be kept to a level normally found in light industry rather than in heavy industrial activities such as coal mining. Have those expectations been fulfilled?

It can be argued that the healthy aspect of working in the nuclear industry is an artefact. It is brought about through the careful selection of people for employment, taking into account both their technical abilities and the state of their health. Radiation workers, by the very nature of their employment, therefore start off with a health advantage which remains throughout their working lives and beyond. Not that radiation workers are unique in that respect: health statistics for the general population show that on average graduates of universities and technical colleges have a much higher life expectancy than those of the same age who go straight from school into full-time employment.

One of the most important series of studies on the health of radiation workers was carried out on the employees, past and present, at the Hanford Works in Richmond, Washington State. The vast nuclear complex at Hanford came into being with the Manhattan Project during World War II (set up to build the first atomic bombs). Hanford was basically a plutonium factory. Nine nuclear reactors were purpose-built to generate plutonium from uranium-238, with the plutonium being dissolved out of the spent reactor fuel in a reprocessing plant. Because of its close association with research and development, the Hanford workforce always had a considerable proportion of people with professional or technical qualifications – just the kind of people with good health statistics.

As a result of regular monitoring of the workers it was known with reasonable accuracy what sort of radiation dose they had received from their work. A study of the deaths from cancer since 1943 indicates that those who were most exposed had a 5 per cent higher rate of cancers than expected. But the data also confirmed that, per unit of radiation exposure, low doses were more damaging than high ones.

31

CHAPTER

⋘ 2 ⋙

Radiation around us

The Solar System is a culmination of billions of years of activity during which energy and matter have been transformed under extreme conditions of gravity, pressure and temperature. These processes resulted in the formation of stars and galaxies. Our Sun is a star which, probably like millions of others, has a system of orbiting planets.

We have therefore inherited naturally occurring elements – both stable and unstable (that is, radioactive) – that came together to form the Sun, Earth and other planets of our Solar System. We are also bombarded with cosmic radiation travelling across the remoteness of space from nuclear events that have taken place in the recent and distant past, possibly on the other side of the galaxy. Together the radioactive elements in the Earth's crust and in the atmosphere, and the high-energy rays from outer space, bathe us perpetually with radiation – natural radiation – which we can

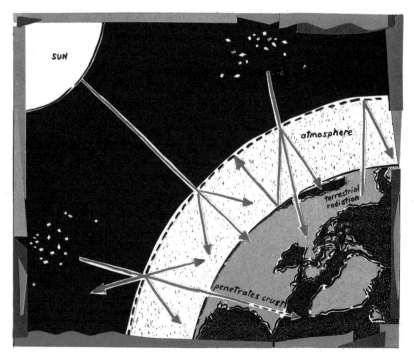

Stars, like the sun, emit radiation. This radiation will penetrate the atmosphere; some of it is deflected and absorbed; some of it gets through to the Earth's surface, that with the highest energy penetrating deep within the Earth itself. Lower energy terrestrial radiation, from radioactive substances like uranium, provides a ground-level exposure to which we are subjected in our daily lives.

never fully avoid. Indeed, as living organisms we have evolved on this Earth against such a background of radiation, only becoming aware of its existence at the end of the last century from the discoveries made by Becquerel, the Curies and other scientists.

Natural background radiation is not uniform, either in time or in space. Over time, the radiation emanating from the Earth has gradually diminished with the constant and inevitable decay of radioactive elements such as uranium and thorium. And while early life forms had to contend with a relatively high radiation background, mammals (including human beings), which evolved much later, came into existence against a natural radiation background that had diminished some 12 times from its levels of 4 billion years ago.

Because life on Earth in all its forms has always been irradiated, can we therefore conclude that radiation at the levels experienced has always been harmless? If it is relatively harmless, the additions resulting from man-made sources such as nuclear power stations must surely be viewed in the same light – because they comprise only a small proportion of the natural background. If, on the other hand, natural background radiation exacts its own toll of human suffering and disease, then we must view any additions – no matter how small – as potentially dangerous.

Cosmic radiation

Originating in the depths of space, cosmic radiation has been bombarding the Earth ever since it was first formed. This radiation is a pot-pourri of different particles and radiation types, some of which have extraordinarily high energies and penetrating powers. The gases in the atmosphere itself are estimated to have a stopping power for ionizing radiation equivalent to a sheet of lead 1 metre (about 3 feet) thick, yet some particles from outer space have been detected a kilometre or more (up to a mile) below the Earth's surface.

A significant amount of cosmic radiation reaching our planet is scattered as it passes through the atmosphere and ultimately loses its energy in a cascade of interactions with airborne particles and gases. As a result, some new radioactive substances are formed, such as the hydrogen isotope tritium, as well as sodium-22 and carbon-14. But the overall effect of the atmosphere is to reduce greatly the amount of cosmic radiation actually reaching the surface of the Earth.

At sea-level, cosmic radiation gives us a yearly dose of just over 0.3 millisieverts. But the dose from this source increases considerably if we live at higher altitudes, doubling at 1,800 metres (5,900 ft) and tripling at around 3,000 metres (9,800 ft). At 4,000 metres (13,100 ft), the altitude of the highest human settlements in the world such as in Ladakh in the Himalayas or in the altiplano of the Andes, the cosmic radiation dose reaches 1.75 millisieverts a year – nearly six times the dose to which one would be exposed at sea-level.

Exposure to cosmic radiation is also signficantly greater for people who spend considerable time flying, such as international travellers and airline crew. At 12,000 metres (39,400 ft), the altitude for intercontinental

(120 km, x 1,000)   spacelab

(20,000m, x 430)

(12,000m, x 170)

(3,000m, x 3)

(1,800m, x 2)

(sea level x 1)

(x 0.1)

(x 0.001)

The levels of cosmic radiation increase rapidly with altitude. As we can see, someone at 3,000 metres will receive 3 times the cosmic radiation compared to someone at sea-level over the same period. Crossing the Atlantic in Concorde, the levels are 430 times greater, but the speed of flight actually results in the radiation dose being some 20 per cent less than that of a subsonic flight.

flights, the cosmic radiation dose goes up nearly 170 times compared to sea-level. Airline crew who may also spend an average of a couple of hours each day flying therefore double their overall radiation dose from all natural sources. Supersonic aircraft such as Concorde are exposed to some 2 times more cosmic radiation while cruising compared to conventional subsonic aircraft, yet because the time to cover a given distance (for instance, across the Atlantic) is less than half, the actual exposure to cosmic radiation is some 20 per cent less. In fact a single flight across the Atlantic at subsonic speeds gives a radiation dose of 0.05 millisieverts, about one-sixth of the yearly dose at sea-level.

As we have already pointed out the unborn child is particularly at risk from low doses of radiation, especially during the first three months of pregnancy. Therefore it would be advisable for pregnant women to take this added risk into consideration before embarking on long haul intercontinental flights, for instance of twelve hours or more.

~~~ Radiation in the ground ~~~

Although we tend to think of radioactive materials as being rare, they are surprisingly plentiful. The Earth contains about one thousand times as much uranium as gold, the uranium for the most part being widely dispersed and only rarely found in concentrations sufficiently high to make mining it a worthwhile proposition. As a result, the radiation produced by the decay of uranium or of thorium – the other main source of terrestrial radiation – is present in measurable quantities almost everywhere. However, such radiation is particularly high in areas where the landscape is dominated by exposed granite, such as in Cornwall in Britain or Maine in the United States, and in monazitic sands which contain high concentrations of thorium. Such sands are found, for instance, in parts of the State of Kerala in India as well as in the state of Espirito Santo in Brazil. In these thorium-rich places exposure rates of up to nearly 30 millisieverts per year have been recorded, therefore giving radiation doses that are ten times higher than the average received elsewhere in the world from all background sources.

Terrestrial radiation impinges on us in different ways, depending on its form and the circumstances in which we encounter it. Somebody living in an area with an average level of background radiation gets a yearly dose of just under 2 millisieverts, with 84 per cent of it coming from terrestrial sources and the remaining 16 per cent from cosmic radiation. On average, one quarter of the terrestrial radiation is in the form of gamma rays emitted from decaying radio-isotopes in the soil and from building materials such as bricks and concrete blocks. Indeed, every second some 55 thousand gamma rays pass through our bodies, a number which appears to be disturbingly large but which has to be viewed in terms of the thousand million million cells in the body with their billions and billions of molecules.

Some regions of the world have high terrestrial levels of background radiation as a result of radioactive mineral deposits. Here we show such 'hot spots' caused by high ground concentrations of uranium and thorium.

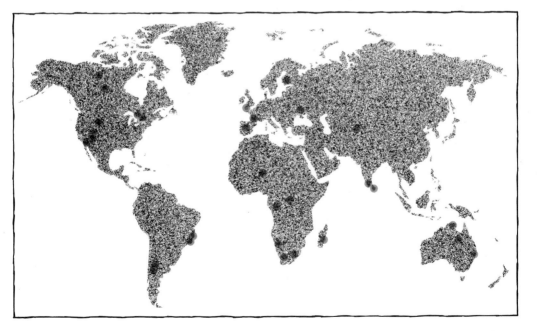

35

Just as altitude and jet-setting affect exposure to cosmic rays, precisely where one lives affects exposure to terrestrial gamma rays. Somebody living along the eastern seaboard of the United States, for example, may receive a gamma dose of no more than 0.15 millisieverts a year, compared to as much as a 9 times greater dose of 1.4 millisieverts for somebody living on the Colorado plateau. There is now evidence that natural background radiation may be responsible for three-quarters of early childhood cancers – amounting to several hundred for every million live births.

Radon gas – increasing concern

In the United States, Britain, Canada and other countries a number of surveys have been carried out of radon levels in homes and public buildings. For the most part the results are reassuring, but in some regions the levels of radon have been sufficiently high to be of concern. Radon is derived from uranium and is in soil and rock. Much of the radon is unable to travel far because of its short half-life. Nevertheless it is able to seep upwards to the surface of the ground where, being denser than air, it accumulates – especially in low-lying areas. It also seeps up into the basements and ground floors of buildings and gets carried into bathrooms with flowing water, gradually building up in showers and baths.

In temperate parts of the world, where the housing is generally not of a very high standard in terms of draught exclusion, the levels of radon inside homes may be as much as eight times higher compared with the outside air. But in energy-efficient homes such those increasingly being built in countries like Sweden with a rigorous winter climate, the levels of radon can rise to 5,000 times or more than the outside levels. Special provisions have to (or should) be made, including forced air circulation, to blow radon out of the house and diminish the risk of contamination.

Radon hot spots

Those of us living in areas that have above average terrestrial gamma radiation levels are also likely to be subjected to high radon levels. The reason is simple enough, because the same uranium and thorium decay

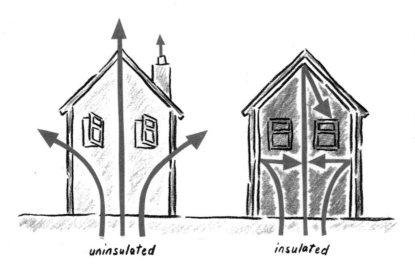

uninsulated   insulated

Radon seeps from the ground. Well-insulated houses tend to accumulate more of this radioactive gas than draughty houses. In certain areas, where there are deposits of radioactive minerals, radon seepage can be a problem.

products are involved in the formation of both gamma rays and radon. As far as human exposure to radon is concerned, the problem is often worsened because areas rich in uranium often have other useful metals such as tin, copper, gold and silver, and the likelihood is that sometime, in the distant or recent past, mining will have occurred.

In parts of Cornwall in western England, where mining for tin and copper has been carried out for centuries, the granite rock is now honeycombed with shafts and galleries, while on the surface mounds of waste tailings have accumulated. Consequently people living close to old mining areas are subjected to much higher radon levels than those found over ground that has been left undisturbed. The NRPB, for instance, found dwellings in Cornwall and Devon that had up to 15 times the radon levels compared to the national average; the survey also revealed a few houses with radon levels at least 50 times higher than the average.

The most extreme instance of radon contamination in the home was in Philadelphia in the United States. The discovery was made after the authorities set out to investigate why the house-owner, Stanley Watras, regularly set off the monitoring alarms at the Limerick nuclear power station were he was employed. They traced the source of contamination to his house, which was found to be constructed directly over an excavated uranium vein. The radon levels were 100,000 becquerels per cubic metre of air. One researcher remarked that 'breathing the air in the house for one day was as risky as smoking 135 packs of cigarettes'.

Radon and lung cancer
It has been known for many years that hard rock miners working underground often have problems with their lungs. As early as the turn of the century, a study revealed that 50 per cent of Czech hardrock miners died of lung cancer. More recent research, this time in uranium mines in Colorado, has revealed similar high mortality rates.

Today it is realized that the likely cause of the high cancer rate is exposure to high radon levels in the mines. Provisions are now made in hardrock underground mining to increase the ventilation of the working galleries so as to sweep out the radon and reduce exposure to the gas.

As a result of increasing concern over the dangers of radon, the United States Enviromental Protection Agency has set the standard of maximum radon levels in homes as 150 becquerels per cubic metre. In contrast the British standard is 400 becquerels per cubic metre – over 2 times as high. Twelve hours a day spent in a house with the American level would give a dose to the lungs each year of 50 millisieverts, or just over 5 millisieverts effective whole-body dose. The risk of contracting fatal lung cancer is therefore increased by approximately 2 per cent for each year's exposure.

Protecting the home from radon
Various strategies can be tried to keep down radon levels in the home. The first, clearly, is to avoid building over ground that has high levels, and the second is to avoid using building materials that are rich in radium and other radioactive substances. Houses can also be built on supports to take the lowest floor above the ground and so prevent seepage into the building. For houses that have already been built and have high radon levels from seepage, various methods have been employed in an attempt to control the

problem, including the installation of a non-permeable membrane under the ground floor and the use of ventilation fans and electrostatic precipitators which take particles out of the air.

Certainly the problem of radon contamination appears to be widespread and serious. At Grand Junction, Colorado, in the mid-1960s local construction firms used the tailings from uranium mines to build houses with the result, as later investigations showed, that levels of radon in some buildings were 1,000 times higher than the natural background level. In 1970 a Colorado paediatrician noticed an increase in cleft palates, hare lips and other congenital defects among children who had been born to parents living in houses constructed from tailings.

A number of building materials have been implicated in causing high radon levels in homes. Alum shales, for instance, were used over several decades in Sweden for making cement, which then found its way into some half a million homes. The alum shales had levels of radium and thorium that exceeded 1,000 becquerels per kilogram (about 450 per lb). Calcium silicate slag, derived from processing phosphate ore, has also been used for concrete manufacture in North America – and that had levels of radioac-

As the bar chart shows some building materials contain far more radioactive minerals than do others. Depending on what materials are used in house construction, the radioactive contamination can vary considerably. Uranium mine tailings used as hardcore ⑩, have a radiation level that is about one hundred times higher than that of portland cement ④, and about 4,500 times that of floor boards ①.

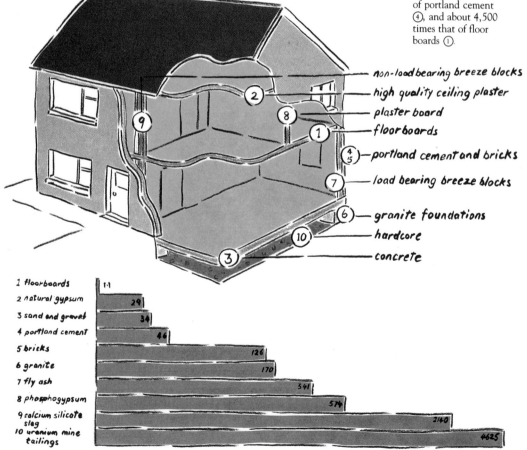

non-load bearing breeze blocks
high quality ceiling plaster
plaster board
floorboards
④⑤ portland cement and bricks
load bearing breeze blocks
⑥ granite foundations
hardcore
concrete

1 floorboards — 1·1
2 natural gypsum — 29
3 sand and gravel — 34
4 portland cement — 46
5 bricks — 126
6 granite — 170
7 fly ash — 341
8 phosphogypsum — 574
9 calcium silicate slag — 2140
10 uranium mine tailings — 4625

tivity exceeding 2,000 becquerels per kilogram (900 per lb). However, the uranium mine tailings were undoubtedly the worst, with more than 4,500 becquerels per kilogram (more than 2,000 per lb).

Phosphogypsum, another by-product of phosphate processing, has been used extensively in West Germany and Japan for making plasterboard and cement. Japan used 3 million tonnes of the material in 1974 alone, and altogether it has been calculated to give an effective dose equivalent – hence a collective whole-body dose – of 300,000 man-sieverts. In effect, people living in houses with such gypsum are expected to have increased their radiation dose by some 30 per cent compared with those living in uncontaminated houses. In that respect, natural gypsum has a radioactive level of merely 29 becquerels per kilogram (13 per lb), and wood, as used in house construction in Finland, of approximately one becquerel per kilogram. Granite in Britain has a level of some 170 becquerels per kilogram (77 per lb).

The most effective way of keeping radon out of buildings is to ventilate the space between the bottom floor and the ground and to cover the walls with plastic materials such as polyvinylchloride (PVC) or epoxy paints. Such methods have been shown to reduce radon infiltration by ten times. Radon coming in with water can be a major problem in certain parts of the world, such as in Finland and parts of the United States. Some water has been found to carry as much as a million becquerels of radon per cubic metre, or even one hundred times that.

In Finland, for instance, radon levels in bathrooms because of the influx with water have been found to be 40 times higher than in the living room of the same house. The problem in cold countries has undoubtedly been aggravated because of the natural desire to save energy and keep heat in the home; as a result, ventilation rates have been cut by more than half since the 1970s and in return the radon levels in houses have tripled. Water used for household purposes is practically free from radon.

If you are concerned about the levels of radon in your area, you should seek the advice of the local authorities.

✦✦✦ Radiation in food ✦✦✦

The foods we eat also contain low levels of radioactive substances, usually because they are grown in areas where background radiation is relatively high. Brazil nuts, for example, contain high levels of thorium and it may be wise to limit the amount you eat. Tea and coffee also tend to contain appreciable levels of radiation, although you would have to drink exceptional quantities to be at risk. Some radioactive elements – particularly radioactive potassium – are found in low levels in all foodstuffs. By and large we are adapted to having such substances decaying radioactively inside us.

The radioactive substances generated by nuclear reactors are not found naturally. If taken in with contaminated food, they mimic natural substances. For instance, radioactive caesium can mimic potassium, an essential substance for the body, and radioactive strontium can mimic calcium and be taken up by bones and teeth. For the body, problems occur as the radioactive substances decay, not simply because of radioactivity but

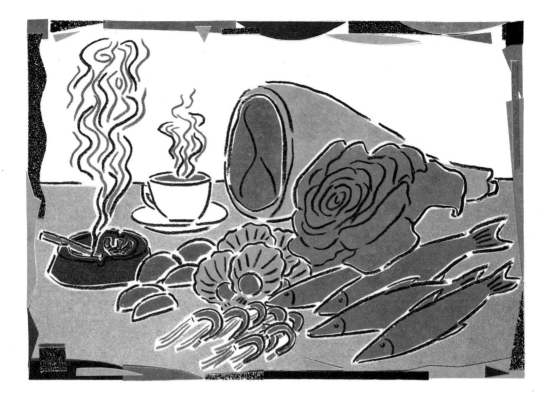

because the substances change their form into totally different elements, which have very different chemical and physical characteristics from the original element. The molecules incorporating those charged elements can no longer serve their precise function in the body and some derangement of biochemical processes is therefore inevitable. However, these effects all take place at the submicroscopic level so that we cannot readily detect them.

Some plants tend to concentrate radioactive isotopes. Tobacco leaves, for instance, have been found to contain low but measurable quantities of the alpha-emitter polonium-210 as well as lead-210. Some scientists have suggested that this contamination with radioactive particles may be responsible either wholly or in part for tobacco's contribution to the incidence of lung cancer.

In fact, the quantities of polonium and other radioactive components that get into the lungs in tobacco smoke are approximately double the levels from alpha-emitters derived from other sources. But, according to the American scientist E.A. Martell, both polonium-210 and lead-210 get taken deep into the lungs as insoluble particles where they lodge and accumulate, whereas other kinds of alpha-emitters are more soluble and get carried away out of the lungs. When an alpha particle is discharged from a decaying polonium atom, it causes intense damage in its vicinity, and Dr Martell and others have suggested that the localized dose delivered to lung tissue by such a 'hot particle' may be as much as 10,000 millisieverts per year. Thus a dose that would appear neglible from a whole-body point of view may be lethal on the minute scale of a lung cell.

Food, drink and tobacco contain natural radioactive substances. Brazil nuts and tea for example tend to have high levels of thorium. Tobacco has relatively high levels of polonium mostly because of the phosphate fertilizer used in growing the plant.

40

Food preservation through irradiation

It is important to distinguish between the presence of unwanted radioactive substances in food and the deliberate use of radiation to preserve it. The purpose of food irradiation is to kill bacteria and other micro-organisms which, if left alive in food, are likely to make it go bad. The technique is thus a form of sterilization. Very high doses are required – of the order of 10,000 grays, equivalent to several million diagnostic X-rays – and the question has arisen, could the food itself undergo harmful changes? The World Health Organization, together with other United Nations agencies, has reviewed the evidence and found that this type of irradiation does not appear to harm food in such a way that it would be dangerous for eating.

Critics of the process point out that irradiation of food destroys its structure and nutritional value by depleting it of vitamins. In addition food irradiation can make food that has gone bad appear to be edible by eliminating the tell-tale signs of decay. Critics are also concerned that some bacteria – such as those that cause botulism – are resistant to irradiation.

Radiation in medicine

Nearly all of us at some stage in our lives have had an X-ray. Until the 1950s they were considered only a blessing. Increasingly, however, the use of X-rays has been associated with an increase in the number of cancer cases. In industrialized countries, X-rays now contribute as much as one-tenth of a person's average natural background dose of radiation.

Every year hundreds of millions of X-ray examinations are carried out, with widely differing doses being given for the same diagnostic procedure. Indeed even within a country from one hospital to another, the dose delivered may vary by a factor of a hundred. The area chosen for irradiation also varies from one place to another, depending on the radiologist, but the aim must be to use the minimum area required to produce a clear picture. In the United States alone, some 300,000 X-ray machines are in current use for medical diagnosis and therapy, as well as for dentistry.

Without question, both patients and staff have benefitted from recent developments in X-ray technology. Special filters to cut out superfluous radiation, faster films which react to lower levels of radiation, better focusing of the X-ray beam and tomography (in which just the image of the desired plane in the body is captured, so cutting out confusing detail) have all contributed to reductions in dose. In Sweden, for instance, the use of tomography increased a hundred fold between 1973 and 1979. As for the dose, conventional X-ray examinations of kidney function – urography – gave 5 times the dose to the skin, 25 times to the ovaries, and 50 times to the testes compared to computerized tomography (better known as a CAT scan).

Radiation doses to the breast – mammography – have also been reduced by as much as 15 times through the use of better equipment and advanced X-ray films. Nevertheless, both in the United States and Sweden, breast examinations more than doubled between 1977 and 1979.

Some kinds of medical diagnosis and treatment depend on the use of radio-isotopes. In the United States, for instance, some 10 to 12 million

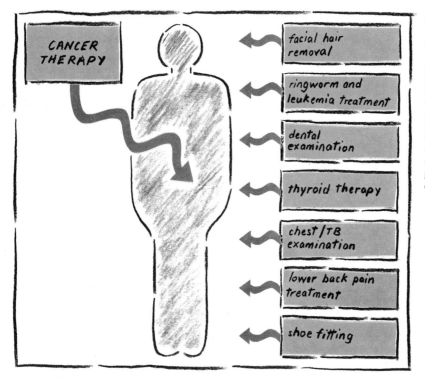

CANCER THERAPY

facial hair removal

ringworm and leukemia treatment

dental examination

thyroid therapy

chest/TB examination

lower back pain treatment

shoe fitting

Since their discovery X-rays have been used extensively for medical diagnosis and treatment as well as for cosmetic purposes. Whereas modern X-ray examinations use relatively low doses of X-rays, cancer therapy, which involves burning the malignant tissues, uses very high doses given to confined areas of the body.

doses are administered each year to check up on such organs as the brain, liver, bones, lungs, thyroid, kidneys and heart, mostly in patients over the age of 44. The diagnostic use of radiopharmaceuticals in the United States represents approximately 20 per cent of the total doses to patients from medical diagnostic radiology. As for those working with such radioactive substances, the annual dose on average lies between 2 and 5 millisieverts, therefore up to one-third of the dose that the NRPB in Britain has recommended should be the annual maximum exposure to radiation for occupationally exposed people.

Because there is some risk associated with diagnostic X-rays, you should always make sure that an X-ray is essential, particularly if children are involved. It is also sensible to insist that every precaution is taken to keep the X-ray dose to a minimum.

X-ray therapy
Very large doses of X-rays, in the range of tens of grays, are given during cancer therapy. Patients survive such doses, but in combination with chemotherapy they may suffer nausea, loss of appetite and temporary loss of hair.

The purpose of the radiation is to destroy cancer cells, either by a beam focused as closely as possible on the tumour or, if the cancer cells have a tendency to pick up a specific chemical, by injecting a highly radioactive version of that chemical. The use of radiation is therefore a trade-off between eradicating the cancer while at the same time increasing the risk of the body developing new cancers.

ᵈᵗᵗ Radiation and the consumer ᵗᵗᵈ

As well as the radon that seeps into homes from the ground and from building materials, it is surprising just how many different sources of radiation there are around us. Who would have thought there could be any risk associated with spectacle lenses, wrist watches and clocks, and even false teeth? Television sets and increasingly other video machines (including word processors) are commonly found in the home and there has certainly been publicity concerning the amount of radiation they emit and whether it is harmful.

Inevitably the cathode-ray tubes used in television sets and other video devices produce some X-rays, but in fact the amount is extremely small and unlikely to have much radiation risk associated with it. The radiation physicist Professor John Gofman, former director of health research at the Lawrence Livermore Laboratory in the United States, calculates that even if someone had the perserverance to watch television for 24 hours a day, over the course of a year the total dose would be no more than 5 millionths of a gray, and therefore barely 4 hundredths of the dose received through natural background radiation.

On the other hand, certain spectacle lenses and porcelain teeth can deliver significant doses. Some optical lenses contain up to 30 per cent uranium or thorium by weight, and 18 per cent is relatively common. Wearing such glasses for 15 hours a day could give a dose of 55 milligrays a year, quite a substantial amount. Uranium is added to the porcelain for making false teeth because it gives a sparkle which mimics the fluorescence of natural teeth. One out of nine people in Britain has artificial porcelain teeth, and according to the NRPB the annual dose equivalent to the individual could be as much as 27 millisieverts – more than 10 times natural background radiation. The NRPB has since recommended that the practice

Many articles in common use such as those shown in the illustration, may give out radiation. New awareness of the risks suggests that in some instances the radiation dose may be excessively high.

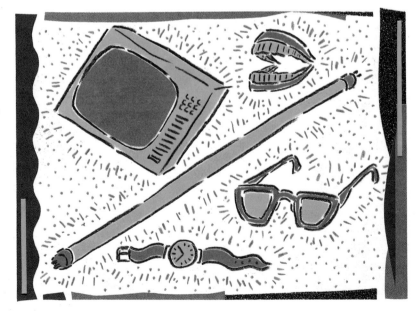

of adding uranium salts to the porcelain should be stopped. Smoke detectors and starters for fluorescent tubes may also contain radioactive substances, but the doses to members of the public are very small.

At risk from radium
According to Professor Gofman, some 23 people in the United States are likely to die each year from cancer brought on through wearing a watch with a luminous dial. The dial is luminous because it is painted with radium and a chemical that fluoresces when irradiated. But far more at risk than the users of such handy devices were those who in the past used to paint the dials. The first luminescent paint factory opened in New Jersey in 1915, hundreds of girls (some no more than 14 years old) being employed to paint dials and even such objects as crucifixes with a mixture of radium and zinc sulphide.

The man who invented the idea, Dr Sabia von Sochocky, insisted that the paint was harmless, but he nonetheless died of cancer at the age of 46, high levels of radium being found in his body. A study of 634 women who worked in the American radium dial painting industry between 1915 and 1929 indicated that the rate of mortality from bone cancer was 80 times higher than expected for women of their age. The girl's habits in applying the radioactive paint had a significant effect on mortality. Before 1924 and the bringing in of regulations concerning how the paint should be applied, the girls used to shape the tips of their brushes with their lips. The cancer rate was found to be more than one hundred times that expected over the period from 1915 to 1924, only dropping dramatically to 9 times the expected rate in those girls who started their employment after some of the risks had been realized. Breast cancer also increased through the work with radium.

By the end of the 1970s, 800,000 radium-dial watches were still in use in Britain. The trend now is to use either tritium or promethium-147 in luminous dials, both of which give a far smaller dose.

Nuclear power and radiation

Nuclear power stations are an obvious source of radiation and a major concern to the public. But even coal-powered power stations release radio-isotopes such as radon in the fly ash that gets discharged into the air and thus into the environment – in addition to all the conventional noxious pollutants such as sulphur dioxide and nitric oxide.

Nevertheless, there are many orders of magnitude between the amount of radioactive waste generated by nuclear power plants and by coal-fired plants. Even though most of the nuclear wastes have to be kept bottled up, the amount that actually gets out into the environment is far greater for a given amount of electricity generated than that from burning fossil fuels.

Uranium mining
The impact of nuclear power on the environment begins with the mining of uranium and the discarding of the tailings (the rock left over after the ore has been extracted). Some 100,000 tonnes of mill tailings are left as a result of producing enough uranium to fuel a one-gigawatt power station for one

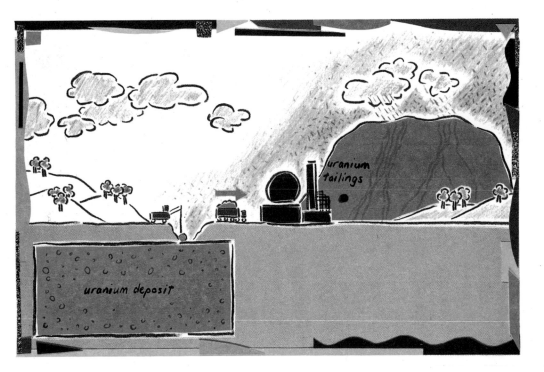

Uranium is usually found in deposits deep underground, where it is out of harms way. Mining the uranium for use in a reactor gives risk to radioactive tailings and debris which can contaminate the environment.

year. They contain 85 per cent of the radioactivity present in the original ore, as well as many other poisonous substances, which before mining were safely locked away below ground. Hundreds of millions of tonnes of tailings now lie on the surface exposed to wind and rain, providing an enormous potential source of cancers and congenital defects.

If we look into the future for the next tens of thousands of years, we find that the nuclear power plants currently operational throughout the world are likely to cause several million premature deaths from lung cancer alone. This probability should make us ensure that uranium mine tailings – as well as those from other hard-rock mining – are dealt with in such a way as to safeguard us from the effects of leaching and seepage.

Geothermal energy (an attractive source of power that uses water heated deep in the ground) is another source of radioactive contamination. This time it is from radon carried up to the surface in the hot waters, giving a dose equivalent to three times that generated by coal-fired power stations for each kilowatt of electricity produced. But the overall contribution to radiation is minimal, because geothermal energy currently provides only one-tenth of one per cent of the world's electricity.

Phosphate rock (used for making artificial fertilizers) is another source of radon, which therefore becomes distibuted wherever commercial farming takes place. But its contribution to radioactive pollution is only about the same as that from geothermal energy.

Atmospheric testing of nuclear weapons
The first nuclear weapon test took place in the New Mexican desert in July 1945. It was a plutonium bomb, with an explosive power equivalent to

45

18,500 tonnes of TNT. The mushroom cloud rose 12,000 metres (40,000 feet) into the atmosphere, and over the next few years gradually showered the ground below with radioactive fall-out.

The next two bombs were those dropped on Hiroshima and Nagasaki in Japan during August 1945. Several hundred thousand people were killed outright, mostly by the blast and the heat but also by a sharp wave of radiation. As with the first test, most of the radioactivity was carried away to fall out over the Earth in the following days, months and years.

More than 1,200 nuclear weapons have been tested since the end of World War II. Initially all were exploded above the ground, although since the 1963 Partial Test Ban Treaty, most have been underground (except those exploded by France, China, India and probably South Africa). The contamination from nuclear explosions has fallen off sharply since the end of atmospheric nuclear testing, although some venting into the atmosphere still takes place. And it is claimed that the French nuclear tests at Muroroa have caused contamination of the sea.

Most of the atmospheric bomb tests took place in the Northern Hemisphere. It is therefore not surprising that most of the fall-out has occurred over the United States, Europe and the Soviet Union. When atmospheric testing was at its peak in the early 1960s, the dose from fall-out over Britain was about 4 per cent of the average natural background dose (but has since fallen by a factor of 8). For the most part, the additional cancers and congenital defects caused by the legacy of the bomb tests will be hard to discern against the normal background of disease in the human population. Nevertheless fall-out has been continually monitored throughout the world, and doses to the population calculated. For instance, one American expert has calculated that nuclear weapon testing up to 1963 may well result in 15,000 additional deaths from cancer over the next few decades among the populations of the heavy fall-out areas of the United States.

Apart from the casualties of Hiroshima and Nagasaki, people were directly affected by nuclear bomb testing. Several thousand were servicemen who witnessed the explosions. Others of the general population suffered as a result of fall-out. Following the Nevada test, for example, high fall-out was detected in the southern and eastern counties of Utah. The rate of leukaemia among children aged between birth and 14 years doubled for those born about 1951, when the testing began, and fell only in those born ten years later when atmospheric testing ceased.

The hazards of nuclear waste
Our exposure to radiation from nuclear power depends very much on where we live and what we do. If we live next to a nuclear plant and work there, our chances of being exposed to radiation are obviously far greater than for someone living in a country which has no such plant. Indeed, living close to a nuclear plant exposes us to radiation in the form of direct gamma rays and some radioactivity in food through isotopes that have escaped from the plant into the environment, albeit through authorized discharges.

The entire nuclear fuel cycle has to be taken into account when estimating collective radiation doses to the public. The fuel cycle describes what happens to uranium all the way through the chain of events that take it out of the ground and into the reactor until the time when it is disposed of. Even

In the upper pie-chart, the main contributor to our yearly radiation dose is seen to be the natural environment around us (67 per cent). Medical radiation diagnosis and treatment is next (11.5 per cent). The routine discharges from nuclear installations on average give us what appears to be an almost negligible 0.1 per cent of the whole. After a nuclear accident, as shown in the lower chart, the situation in the worst affected areas can be completely reversed, with the greatest contributor to the yearly dose being radioactive fall-out. Natural background radiation then becomes by comparison, a relatively minor source.

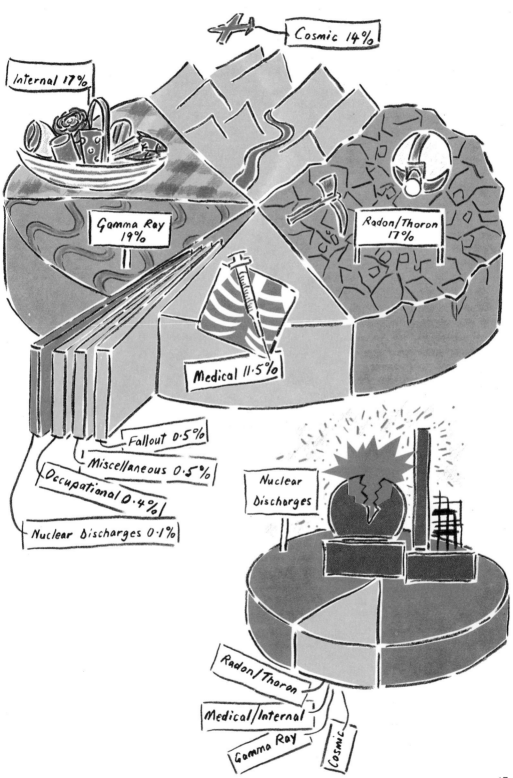

Cosmic 14%

Internal 17%

Gamma Ray 19%

Radon/Thoron 17%

Medical 11.5%

Fallout 0.5%

Miscellaneous 0.5%

Occupational 0.4%

Nuclear Discharges 0.1%

Nuclear Discharges

Radon/Thoron

Medical/Internal

Gamma Ray

Cosmic

after disposal, whether in long-term storage on the surface or buried in some deep repository, some release of radioactive substances into the environment may occur and give future generations a measurable radiation dose.

Nuclear power generates a staggering quantity of radioactive substances, which as far as is economically and practically possible have to be kept bottled up and away from the living environment. One large reactor, generating one gigawatt of electricity per year, has its fuel for one year's operation derived from 96,000 tonnes of rock and shale. Most of this is left behind as tailings after the extraction of the uranium, and most of the radioactivity remains in the tailings. Indeed, whereas the fresh fuel for a year's electricity generation in one gigawatt of nuclear power contains some 10 curies of radioactivity, the tailings contain 67 curies and therefore seven times as much.

By the end of the century the quantities of tailings from uranium mining operations is likely to be in the range of 500 million tonnes. If precautions are not taken to cover the waste mine debris and prevent leaching, the collective dose could reach several thousand person-sieverts for every gigawatt of electricity produced over the course of a year – an amount as large as the collective radiation dose that would accrue from the fly-ash of 1,000 large coal-fired electricity plants.

Even that quantity of radiation from the tailings – some 335,000 curies overall – pales into insignificance compared to the quantities generated during the operation of a nuclear power reactor. After a year in the reactor at full power, the fuel produces some 5 billion curies, which is 79 million times more than that originally found in the ore.

The physical half-lives of many of the fission products in the spent fuel can be measured in seconds or days rather than months or years, and the radioactivity falls away rapidly once the fuel is out of the reactor. To minimize human exposure, the spent fuel is first extracted from the reactor by remote control and then placed under water in a special cooling pond. The water acts as shielding against the barrage of radiation emanating from the fuel and helps to cool it. In fact considerable heat is generated by the fission products in the fuel when first extracted from the reactor.

The 180 million curies in each tonne of fuel from a modern pressurized water reactor (PWR) drops to 4.64 million curies after 150 days, to 693,000 curies after a year and finally after 10,000 years to 470 curies. Some 30 tonnes of uranium fuel are required for each year's PWR operation, and therefore even after 10,000 years the radioactivity in the fuel is nearly 200 times greater than in the ore from which the fuel was extracted.

After half a year's cooling, dangerous alpha emitters such as plutonium, neptunium, and americium comprise no more than 3 per cent of the total radioactivity. However, as the shorter-lived fission products (including substances such as caesium-137, strontium-90 and iodine-131) decay away, the proportion of the longer-lived alpha emitters increases until after 10,000 years it reaches 96 per cent.

The spent fuel, if it were kept intact for 10,000 years, would still be lethal from radioactivity; indeed one kilogram of such fuel would contain 18 million times more radioactivity than the 1,000 becquerels per kilogram of lamb which the British Government laid down as the upper limit considered fit for human consumption following the accident at Chernobyl and the fall-out of radioactive caesium over Britain.

The nuclear industry is under an immense obligation to ensure that the radioactive waste from spent fuel is kept clear of the living environment for many thousands of years. Just what method will be favoured in the long term remains to be seen, and scientists are looking into the safety of different ways of disposal, including dropping canisters of waste several thousand metres into what are considered stable geological rock formations, whether on land or under the seabed. They have to be sure that the site chosen will remain clear of major movements of the Earth, including the shifting of the continental plates, earthquakes and volcanic activity.

UNSCEAR – the United Nations Scientific Committee on the Effects of Atomic Radiation – takes the view that scientists will solve the problems of nuclear waste disposal and that the dose contribution over the next few thousand years will be negligible, certainly no more than 0.1 per cent of the total dose commitment from nuclear power.

In the meantime, certain countries with nuclear power treat the spent fuel chemically in order to extract plutonium and uranium. The reprocessing of spent fuel dissolves out all the nuclear waste fission products, which are then channelled into stainless steel tanks that have to be kept cool, to counteract the heat from the decaying radionuclides. Inevitably the reprocessing of spent fuel leads to the escape of certain radioactive gases such as krypton-85 and water vapour containing tritium. Various other nuclear wastes accumulate in sludges and resins as a result of the treatment, and have to be packaged and conditioned so as not to contaminate the environment. Some wastes are discharged into waterways and into the sea, opening up biological pathways by which they can come back to human beings.

CHAPTER

3

Nuclear power and its future in the world

At the end of World War II, many scientists were keen to develop a peaceful use for the atom. What better way could there be of using the energy of nuclear fission than to generate electricity? In a bout of undisguised euphoria, several scientists and engineers pronounced that atomic energy would solve mankind's energy problems for all time. Electricity, said some, would be too cheap to meter.

In April 1947 the chairman of the newly established US Atomic Energy Commission told an audience of top-ranking Americans that the small cylinder of shining metal he was holding in his hand contained 'power we can release and control, that equals the burning of 2,500 tons of coal. Probably the most important decisions we will ever make in our history as a nation concerns the use we will make of uranium.'

The Soviets also saw great hope for themselves and mankind in nuclear power. In September 1949 they announced that they would use uranium-burning stations to produce power, and nuclear explosives to 'move unwanted mountains, alter the course of great rivers, irrigate deserts and make them bloom'.

The reality
Just what has happened to all those dreams? In the United States, the Soviet Union, Britain, Canada and France, the fledgling nuclear industries began to build a series of nuclear power stations based on different designs and by no means all of them purely peaceful in intent. Indeed, plutonium is a by-product of reactor operation and if extracted from the reactor fuel (where it has formed) and then concentrated, it makes an extremely effective explosive device. Aside from Canada, all the other countries developing nuclear power in the 1950s and 1960s did so with ambivalent motives.

Also the sharing of costs between the civilian sector and the military gave nuclear power a seeming economic advantage over most conventional forms of electricity generation (the exception being pollution-free hydro-electricity). But the reality, appreciated as early as the 1950s by the head of Britain's nuclear power programme, Lord Hinton, was that nuclear power could not compete economically with coal as a fuel. That reality has remained to this day, despite persistent statements to the contrary by government ministers and the nuclear industry itself.

The figures speak for themselves. In the 1970s, when ordering of new nuclear power stations was rising in leaps and bounds, it was generally forecast that globally as many as 4,500 large (approximately one gigawatt in size) nuclear plants would be in operation by the year 2000. This would be enough to provide for double the world's 1987 electricity capacity, and 17 times the current nuclear capacity. Present forecasts are down by a factor of nine on the 1970s figure, and even this is likely to be a conservative reduction.

Perhaps the best indicator of the fortunes of nuclear power must be the United States, where the process of building up a programme of nuclear power stations actually began. By 1986 the country had 93 operating nuclear power stations capable of delivering 78,000 megawatts of electricity, with 26 other plants under construction (to provide an additional capacity of 29,000 megawatts) – surely the hallmarks of a succesful industry. However, since 1977 not one new nuclear power station has been ordered and one hundred that had been ordered since 1973 have been cancelled. Those that have survived the axe have taken ten years or more to complete as new safety requirements have been demanded, and their costs have escalated accordingly.

In the chain reaction, a neutron crashes into a fissile uranium atom, splitting it into two more or less equal halves with the release of energy in the form of heat, gamma rays and several neutrons.

Counting the cost

One of the most spectacular rises in price was for five nuclear plants ordered by the Washington Power Supply System, which were originally estimated to cost $4,000 million in the early 1970s. Within a decade the costs had risen to $26,000 million. This had the effect of bankrupting many of the local authorities that had invested in the project and three of the five reactors were moth-balled, unlikely ever to be finished.

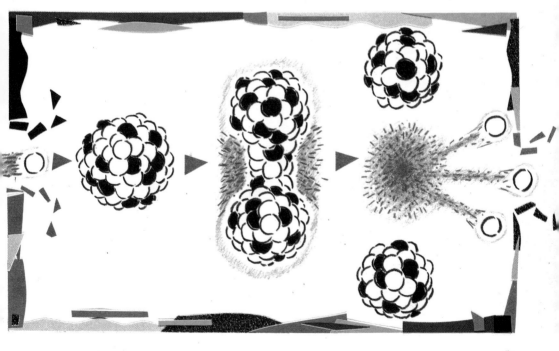

Some have ascribed the fall in the fortunes of nuclear power to the accident at the Three Mile Island reactor in March 1979, which left a clean-up bill of more than one billion dollars and scores of local citizens on the verge of nervous breakdowns. Yet even before that accident, concern had been growing over the safety of reactors in the United States. The Nuclear Regulatory Commission had begun demanding that a host of new safety measures be implemented before licences to operate would be issued. Many reactors had to be re-designed and back-up safety systems fitted retrospectively during the course of construction. As was shown in a number of studies, nuclear power was becoming far more costly as a source of electricity compared with coal even when coal-fired stations had to comply with ever-more stringent pollution regulations. Public utilities, which in the United States are privately-owned facilities for electricity generation, began to discover the virtues of energy conservation measures. In some parts of the country – Washington State, for instance – they exhorted their customers to save electricity rather than consume more, a fundamental switch in thinking from the growth for growth's sake mentality of the 1960s.

Apart from the United States, the country with the most nuclear reactors in operation is France. Instituted in 1973 the French nuclear power programme consisted of a production line manufacture of Westinghouse pressurized water reactors, the aim being to embark on the construction of five to six new reactors each year with some six years being taken to complete each one. That programme has come to fruition, as planned, and at present some 70 per cent of France's electricity is generated by nuclear power stations, there being some 50 units connected to the grid with some 20 others under construction.

The programme planners anticipated an annual growth in electricity consumption of 7 per cent per year – that is, a doubling every decade. But that growth rate has not occurred, and France is moving rapidly to the time when it will have ten or more nuclear power stations surplus to its needs. In response, since 1984 the French government has progressively reduced the construction programme from six to two and now to one firm order per annum.

Nuclear power stations generate electricity. When that electricity is used for heating houses, not only is it inefficient in energy terms because of the large heat losses to the environment during its generation – losses of more than 60 per cent – but it is expensive too. Indeed, as France's electricity board has discovered to its cost, when electricity is used for domestic heating there is enormous fluctuation in demand from week to week, with nearly half the nation's electricity generating capacity having to remain idle one week and in use the next.

The next largest nuclear power programme is in the Soviet Union, which will surpass France's overall generating capacity if the projected plans go ahead. By the beginning of 1986, the Soviet Union had 51 reactors connected to the grid with a total generating capacity of just under 28,000 megawatts. However 34 more reactors are under construction, with a total generating capacity of 32,000 megawatts. As in France, the great majority of the new plants being built are pressurised water reactors. Nevertheless the Soviet Union is building 7 more large reactors of the same type as the Chernobyl RBMK which exploded in April 1986, and has brought back into operation all the three remaining RBMKs at the Chernobyl site,

A nuclear reactor consists basically of a core containing fuel which undergoes fission and generates heat. The heat is taken away by circulating coolant which operates a turbine. The end result is the generation of electricity.

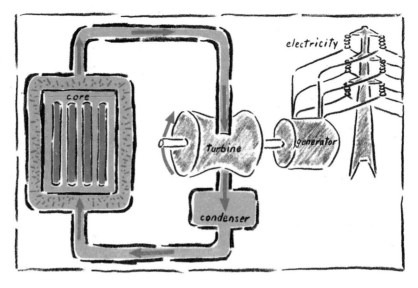

leaving the destroyed number 4 reactor encased in a mausoleum of concrete. Altogether the Soviet Union has 27 RBMKs still in operation, generating 56 per cent of the country's nuclear electricity.

The other industrialized nation with a sizeable nuclear power programme is Japan, which by 1986 had 33 reactors installed, with a capacity of some 24,000 megawatts. It then had another 11 plants capable of generating 10,000 megawatts under construction. Despite the impact of Chernobyl on public opinion in Japan, the government was pushing ahead for at least 40 per cent of electricity to be nuclear generated by the year 2000. Particular precautions were being taken against seismic shocks from earthquakes at the reactor sites.

West Germany has a relatively large nuclear programme, with 19 reactors in operation capable of generating some 16,500 megawatts of electricity, and it has another 6 reactors under construction, adding another 6,600 megawatts to the system.

Britain, which ventured into nuclear power early so as to obtain plutonium for its weapons programme, has a number of relatively small reactors in operation, thus boosting the numbers in return for a relatively small generating capacity. Altogether Britain has 38 operating reactors, capable of generating some 10,000 megawatts. Another 5 units are under construction, four of which are gas-cooled like most of the others. The latest at Sizewell in Suffolk is a large pressurized water reactor, for which planning permission was granted by the government in March 1987.

More than 30 countries have now embarked on nuclear power programmes. Some of these are extensive, others are like that of Mexico – originally ambitious but now pared right down as the economic realities of paying for such imported technology have hit home. Mexico, for instance, ordered 20 reactors in the early 1970s, but has now restricted itself to two, while both Brazil and Argentina have also cut back on their plans. The Philippines had one plant under construction, but on coming to office President Aquino brought all work on the reactor to a standstill.

53

China, meanwhile, has asked France to build a pressurized water reactor at Daya Bay, across the border from Hong Kong. Construction has now begun, despite the concern of the population in the British colony, who are worried about safety and radioactive pollution. In 1986, following the Chernobyl accident, China announced that it was cancelling eight of another ten plants planned.

Yugoslavia has also announced that it will not be adding in the near future to the 600-megawatt plant it has in operation, and Austria, which had completed construction of a reactor at Zwentendorf, made it clear that it would be abiding by a public referendum on nuclear power in which the majority voted against it. The Zwentendorf plant will therefore not be fuelled.

Sweden obtains 50 per cent of its electricity from nuclear power and the remainder from hydro-electric plants. In a referendum held in 1980, the Swedes voted for the complete phasing out of nuclear power from the country's generation system by the year 2010. The government had hoped for a change of heart, but the accident at Chernobyl further entrenched public opinion. (Parts of Sweden received high levels of fall-out from the accident in the Ukraine.)

Altogether in the world, some 375 reactors are now connected to the electricity grid with another 156 in the process of construction. At best nuclear power plants have an operating lifetime of some 30 to 35 years, and already a number of the earliest power-generating reactors are reaching the end of their lives. Unless there is a new spurt in reactor ordering it would seem that the population of reactors will fall early in the next century. Indeed, nuclear power is limited in providing the world with energy. Compared for instance with traditional fuels, whether they be firewood, cattle dung, or the ubiquitous fossil fuels, nuclear power lacks flexibility. And the economic realities of deploying it make it an unlikely form of energy for the vast majority of people now or in the foreseeable future.

How reactors work

Albert Einstein predicted that enormous quantities of energy would be released when matter lost bits of mass. That is precisely what happens in a nuclear fission reaction. Indeed, every time a uranium or plutonium atom splits into two more-or-less equal-sized new atoms (which are themselves radioactive), energy is released in the form of powerful gamma rays, high-velocity neutrons and intense heat. In an atomic bomb, all the fissile material is made to deliver as much energy as possible in a few millionths of a second. In a nuclear reactor, however, the same amount of energy is released over several months in a controlled way. The energy is used to heat up water until it becomes superheated steam, just as in a conventional power station. The high-pressure steam then spins a turbine, which is linked to a generator for producing electricity. Thus the principal difference between a nuclear power station and an ordinary one is merely the source of the heat used to boil water.

Types of reactors

When nuclear physicists and engineers first began to design reactors, they found themselves confronted with a number of basic possibilities. In the end the design was determined by the reactor's function. As a result, the first reactors to be built, such as the N-reactors at Hanford in Washington State, or the gas-cooled Magnox reactors in Britain and France, had as their primary purpose the production of plutonium for weapon-making.

The Magnox types had a distinct advantage over the earlier N-reactors in that they were dual-purpose: thus they also generated electricity, and therefore offset some of the cost of plutonium production. On the other hand, the pressurized water reactor – the PWR – was originally designed to power nuclear submarines, which required a compact, high-power reactor that could be housed within the hull of a sea-going vessel.

After President Eisenhower's Atoms for Peace Programme of the mid-1950s, the race was on to develop nuclear reactors that could be used to generate electricity for civilian use. The Westinghouse Company, which had developed the PWR for nuclear submarines, then came up with the Shippingport reactor. This was a prototype small, land-based version which came into operation in 1958 – having taken only three years to build, therefore a remarkably short time.

PWRs have since proved to be the world's most popular design of nuclear reactor. Currently some 190 of them are in operation, the majority in the United States with 67, followed by France with 40, the Soviet Union with 19 and West Germany with 10. In addition to those in operation, there are 115 under construction and more than 70 in the planning stage. One reason for the popularity of PWRs is that most of its essential components, including the reactor pressure vessel, steam generator and turbines, can be manufactured in a factory rather than on site. Production in a factory has

The most popular reactor in the world is the PWR (Pressurized Water Reactor). Water under pressure takes heat from the nuclear fuel and exchanges it with water in a separate circuit which, because it is under much less pressure, can boil and generate steam. Steam works the turbine. The PWR has a strong steel pressure vessel; control rods can be dropped into the core to stop the chain reaction.

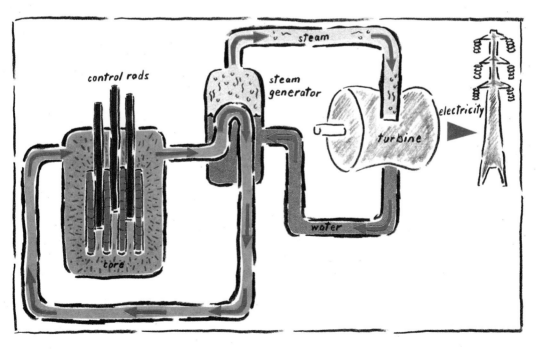

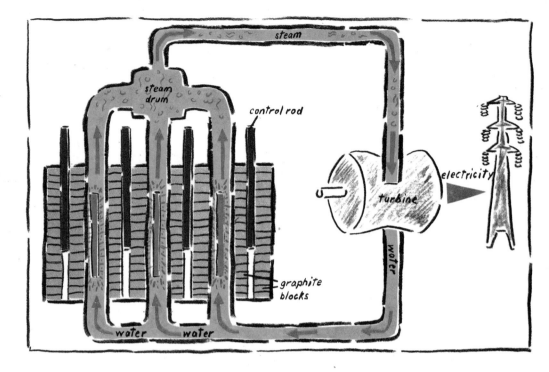

steam

steam drum

control rod

turbine

electricity

graphite blocks

water

water

water

the advantage that it reduces both the overall cost of the complete nuclear plant, as well as the time taken for construction.

The British designed gas-cooled reactors, the Magnox and the Advanced Gas Reactors (AGRs), have to be built on site. The prime reason is that the pressure vessel (which is fabricated from steel in a PWR) in the current version of the gas-cooled reactors is made of reinforced concrete. Britain's main electricity producer, the Central Electricity Generating Board, has now favoured the PWR and intends to build a series of such reactors.

The boiling water reactor (BWR), which was also developed in the United States in the 1950s, is another type to have attracted clients throughout the industrialized world. The United States now has 32 BWRs in operation and another 6 being built. West Germany has 7, Japan 16, Sweden 9 and Taiwan 4 BWRs, with Japan constructing another 5. Throughout the world 79 BWRs are in commission with another 15 under construction. In a PWR, the water used to convey the heat out of the core is under such pressure – some 170 atmospheres – that it remains liquid and does not boil. In a BWR, as the name denotes, the water is under less pressure and therefore does boil. The advantage of the BWR is that the boiling water can be used immediately to spin the turbogenerator, whereas the PWR has to have a secondary cooling circuit at a lower pressure in which the steam is raised for working the turbine.

Both the PWR and BWR use highly purified, but otherwise normal, water, which is therefore designated 'light water'. Other reactors, such as Canada's CANDU type or Britain's Steam Generating Heavy Water Reactor (SGHWR), use heavy water that is highly enriched with deuterium. Such heavy water reactors are similar to the Soviet RBMK type in that,

The RBMK – a reactor such as that used in the Soviet Union at Chernobyl – has a graphite moderator with pressure tubes containing fuel and water. The water boils to steam in the upper part of the tubes and after collecting in a steam drum goes to work the turbine. The control rods slip down between the graphite blocks.

instead of having a single pressure vessel (as in a PWR), they use a series of pressure tubes. Both the CANDU and SGHWR reactors have secondary coolant circuits for generating steam, whereas the RBMK allows steam to build up in the upper half of the pressure tubes from where it passes to a steam drum and then to the turbogenerators. The pressure-tube system is basically a modular one which enables the reactors to be scaled-up without running into problems regarding the construction and strength of the pressure vessel.

Breeder reactors

Nuclear physicists discovered soon after construction of the first reactor that uranium-238, the heavy isotope of natural uranium, could capture a neutron and become the new element plutonium. Because plutonium undergoes nuclear fission when bombarded with neutrons, they recognized that the near-ideal design of a reactor would be one in which as much plutonium was created as uranium was consumed. Indeed, in principle, such a reactor could even produce a surplus of fissile material that could then be used to fuel another reactor.

Such breeding of fuel is not making something out of nothing. On the contrary, if uranium-238 (which makes up more than 99 per cent of all natural uranium) did not transform into plutonium, then the fissioning of uranium would be limited just to the 0.7 per cent of the fissile isotope uranium-235. The breeding of plutonium also depends on the fortuitous circumstance that when uranium-235 undergoes fission it releases several neutrons. One of these neutrons is required to sustain the nuclear chain reaction by fissioning another uranium-235 atom. The remaining neutron(s) either escape entirely from the reactor, or get absorbed by some material within it. If that material is uranium-238, some plutonium will be 'bred'. In fact, nearly all reactor systems, whether they are light water reactors, heavy water reactors or gas-cooled reactors, have considerable

A fast breeder reactor has no moderator so the neutrons remain at high speed. The fuel is densely packed and enriched with plutonium. The coolant is liquid metallic sodium and after an intermediate sodium circuit, steam is generated in a heat exchanger to work the turbine. The core is surrounded by an uranium blanket so that surplus neutrons breed more plutonium.

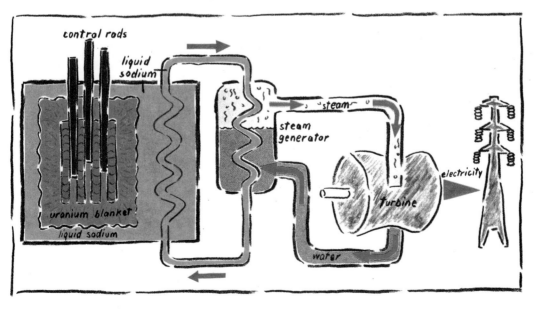

quantities of uranium-238 in the fuel and therefore some plutonium is created which can later be extracted. Indeed it is that property of breeding which is exploited in designing dual-purpose plutonium and electricity production reactors such as Magnox.

However, there is a way of increasing the amount of breeding, and that is by surrounding the nuclear core of the reactor with a blanket of uranium that is almost entirely uranium-238. Thus, any neutrons that escape from the fissioning process in the core pass into the blanket where the chances are high that plutonium will be formed. Reactors using this type of design are known as breeder reactors.

But there is another outstanding feature of breeder reactors: they do not have a 'moderator' in the core. When scientists were first trying to develop a chain reaction, they discovered that the chances of getting one uranium fission to lead to another were much improved if the neutrons flying out from the disintegrating nucleus could be slowed down without being absorbed in the process. Materials that do this slowing down are called moderators. The best ones proved to be hydrogen, deuterium and carbon, and they were used in the form of light or heavy water or, in the case of carbon, as graphite. In fact no moderator is perfect, and there is always some trade-off between a moderator's ability to slow down neutrons to the ideal speed for fissioning uranium and their characteristic of absorbing neutrons. If they absorb too many, they in effect stifle the chain reaction.

Scientists also discovered that the slowed-down neutrons – called thermal neutrons – are not as effective as more energetic ones in being absorbed by uranium-238. Therefore, although the fissioning of uranium-235 is enhanced by slowed-down thermal neutrons, plutonium breeding from uranium-238 is reduced. The compromise in the fast breeder reactor is to do away with the moderator but instead increase the percentage of fissile

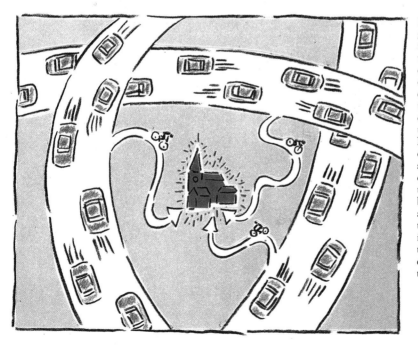

In nuclear power generation the use of a moderator, such as water or graphite, slows down the neutrons escaping from a disintegrating nucleus, thus increasing the chances of splitting a uranium atom. Neutrons when first emitted travel at high speeds (the cars) and easily miss the uranium target (the village). By being forced to travel at much slower speeds the neutrons become ideal for fission and like the slow moving cyclists can arrive at their destination.

material (plutonium) in the fuel. A fast reactor therefore has fuel enriched to 15 per cent or more compared to the 3.5 per cent maximum of conventional thermal reactor systems such as PWRs.

Many materials will absorb neutrons. Steel is an effective absorber, as is the element known as boron. Some fission products generated during the chain reaction, such as xenon-135, are very potent neutron absorbers and they tend to poison the chain reaction. Luckily for the reactor designers, xenon-135 has a half-life of just over 9 hours and therefore it does not accumulate.

It is this property of certain materials to absorb neutrons that is exploited in shutting reactors down. In general highly absorbent (in terms of neutrons) metal rods are made to slide between the fuel rods – which are normally stacked vertically, or sometimes horizontally, as in the CANDU system. In emergencies, the neutron-absorbing rods – known as control rods – are driven or dropped as quickly as possible into the core. Free-flying neutrons are then mopped up and the chain reaction quickly withers away. It starts up again when the control rods are pulled out of the reactor core.

Enriched uranium

The prime reason a fast reactor needs highly enriched fuel is because of the difference between fast and slow neutrons. A fast neutron has 100 million times more energy than a slow thermal neutron, and moves so fast through the core that it is likely to escape without being captured by the nucleus of a fissile atom. Indeed a slow neutron has at least a 100-times better chance of absorption than a fast neutron.

However, enriched uranium does not exist naturally and has to be created by an energy-costly process. The first enrichment plant to be built, at Oak Ridge in Tennessee, worked on the principle of diffusion of gases through a membrane. The natural uranium, with a content of 0.7 per cent uranium-235 and 99.3 per cent uranium-238, was first converted into a highly corrosive, toxic gas and then pumped under pressure through a porous membrane. The slightly heavier uranium-238 tended to go through the membrane less easily than the smaller uranium-235. Thus after many stages, a gradual separation of the two isotopes was achieved, producing one gas rich in uranium-235 and the other depleted of this fissile isotope. The original purpose of the enrichment plant was purely military, the uranium-235 recovered from the process being sent to Los Alamos in New Mexico for making into the bomb that devastated Hiroshima.

Countries such as Britain and France, which wanted to develop their own nuclear weapons after World War II, did not have the enormous resources of the United States. They found the building of atomic reactors for plutonium production a cheaper way of getting fissile material for bomb-making than enriching uranium. Indeed, vast quantities of electricity for the pumps were required in the gaseous diffusion plant and neither Britain nor France could match the cheap, surface-mined coal that the United States had in plentiful supply for electricity generation.

The lack of any enrichment facility in Europe in the post-war era also determined the design of the first nuclear power plants built in the 1950s in Britain and a little later in France. The fuel had to be manufactured from natural uranium with its very low uranium-235 content, and that meant using an efficient moderator. Graphite, with its lattice-work of carbon

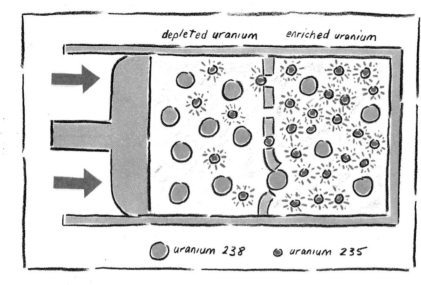

depleted uranium   enriched uranium

uranium 238   ● uranium 235

To enrich nuclear fuel with uranium 235, one method is to pump uranium hexafluoride gas through a membrane; the smaller uranium 235 passes through more easily than the larger uranium 238. After many stages the uranium is enriched to the desired level with uranium 235.

atoms, fitted the bill and was not only used in the original plutonium piles at Windscale in Cumbria, but also in the Magnox power stations that followed, and finally in the advanced gas reactors now operating in Britain.

Because of the high concentration of uranium-238 in the natural uranium used in Magnox reactors, plutonium production is enhanced. Fast breeder reactors, with their blanket of depleted uranium rich in the 238-isotope surrounding the core, are also excellent for the production of high-quality plutonium. PWRs with their enriched fuel generate less plutonium compared with the natural uranium reactors for a given output of electricity. Nevertheless even in a PWR a considerable quantity of plutonium is produced, some of which takes part in the chain reactions. When the reactor is in full operation, approximately 30 per cent of the energy released comes from plutonium fissionings and the remaining 70 per cent from uranium-235.

Reactors using natural uranium fuel are far more bulky than those with enriched fuel. A Magnox reactor needs some 340 tonnes of natural uranium fuel to generate one gigawatt of power over a year, compared with 30 tonnes of enriched fuel for PWRs and 4 to 5 tonnes for a fast reactor. Today nobody favours building a natural uranium reactor because of the high cost of construction.

The gaseous diffusion method of enriching uranium still holds sway in France at Tricastin, where four PWRs generate electricity for a large enrichment facility. It is also used in the United States and the Soviet Union. Britain, having developed a gaseous diffusion plant at Capenhurst during the late 1950s, has now developed an alternative method of enrichment based on a cascade of ultracentrifuges each spinning at a 100,000 revolutions per minute.

The advantage of ultracentrifuges is their better efficiency and they consume far less electricity compared with diffusion. Other potentially more efficient methods in the pipeline include laser enrichment. The danger is that such methods will enable countries to enrich uranium for bomb-making.

Different reactor systems

From a design point of view, the advantage of light water reactors is that the water circulating through the core doubles up as both moderator and heat extractor. The hydrogen atoms in water (H_2O) are very nearly the same size as the neutrons coming off the disintegrating uranium, and therefore just as a billiard ball will slow down or stop when colliding with another billiard ball, but will bounce with most of its energy intact off the heavy sides of the table, so a neutron is best slowed down by hydrogen atoms. However, hydrogen readily absorbs neutrons to become deuterium or heavy hydrogen, and in a reactor that is using natural uranium this brings the chain reaction rapidly to a close. Light or ordinary water can therefore be used only in reactors that employ enriched uranium.

Deuterium (heavy hydrogen) is double the mass of ordinary hydrogen, and is thus less effective in slowing down neutrons to thermal speeds, but its absorption of neutrons is minimal. As long as enough of it is used, heavy water can therefore serve as moderator and coolant in reactors that employ natural uranium as fuel. The Canadian CANDU reactor uses heavy water, as does Britain's Steam Generating Heavy Water prototype reactor, although the latter uses a mixed system with heavy water purely as moderator and light water coursing over the fuel inside pressure tubes as coolant. Some enrichment of fuel is therefore needed for the SGHWR.

Both Britain and France built a series of Magnox reactors for plutonium production in the 1950s and 1960s, electricity initially being a by-product but in later versions the primary purpose. Indeed there is a trade-off between plutonium production and electricity generation insofar as the most economic way to generate electricity is to get as much as possible out of the fuel before having to replace it.

The Magnox reactors have graphite blocks as the moderator, with the fuel and control rods sliding through channels within the graphite. The graphite, being immobile and solid, cannot therefore function as a coolant to take heat out of the core. Instead, carbon dioxide gas under pressure is used. In heat exchangers, the gas gives up its heat to water passing through thousands of boiler tubes, and the resulting steam is used to power the turbines.

Advanced gas reactors (AGRs) work on fundamentally the same principle as the Magnox, graphite again serving as moderator and carbon dioxide gas as coolant. However, whereas the first Magnox reactors had a steel pressure vessel to hold the core together and keep in the circulating gas, AGRs – like the later Magnox – use a vast reinforced concrete pressure vessel. Because of its strength, the pressure vessel in the AGRs doubles up as a containment structure to keep in the highly radioactive fission products should there be an accident inside the reactor. And like light water reactors, AGRs use enriched fuel which is in ceramic oxide form, giving it a higher melting point than the uranium metal fuel used in a Magnox.

The fuel, either in its metallic form or more usually today as an oxide, is clad in material which holds it together and gives it strength. The cladding also serves to hold in the fission products, including gases, as they are formed. Magnox fuel is clad in a magnesium alloy which has the advantage that it is comparatively strong and yet it does not have great neutron-absorbing properties. AGRs, like fast reactors, use special stainless steel cladding, with the fuel in the form of small-diameter metre-long pins held together in bundles. Light water reactors use a zirconium alloy for cladding, the advantage again being that not too many neutrons are absorbed and the cladding offers strength.

The Chernobyl type RBMK was dubbed a hybrid, chimaeric reactor after the accident. Yet all reactors utilize a combination of different materials in their operation. In fact, the RBMK uses graphite as moderator and ordinary water as coolant, running through a series of vertical boiler tubes which like the fuel cladding are fabricated from zircalloy. The water boils in the upper half of the tubes and therefore, like the boiling water reactor, only one coolant circuit is required. The RBMK also uses enriched fuel.

Another gas-cooled reactor was designed for operating at high temperatures. The High Temperature Reactor (HTR) therefore uses graphite as moderator but helium instead of carbon dioxide as coolant gas. In fact carbon dioxide becomes very corrosive for graphite at high temperatures. Helium, on the other hand, is an inert gas. Its main disadvantage is that it is more expensive.

The HTR uses highly enriched fuel, as high as 93 per cent in uranium-235, in the form of graphite coated spheres. Breeding is achieved by inter-dispersing the fuel with another fertile material, thorium-232. Instead of transforming into plutonium on absorbing a neutron, thorium converts into uranium-233 (which is fissile, like uranium-235).

Apart from its potential fuel-breeding characteristics, another hoped-for advantage of the HTR is that the high-temperature coolant gas can be used directly to power a gas turbine, or its heat used as 'process' heat in industry. However, the helium gas has the unfortunate characteristic of cleansing moving parts of any lubricants. A small prototype HTR – the Dragon reactor – has been tested in Britain. Several HTRs have also been built in West Germany and the United States. The latest in Germany, the Hamm HTR, which was due to go into operation in 1986, was shut down after a leak which coincided with the Chernobyl accident. It has since started up.

Five fast reactors of various sizes are in operation in the world: three in the Soviet Union, one in Britain and one in France. Several others are under construction, particularly in West Germany and Japan. The largest, and the one with the greatest commercial pretensions, is France's 1,300-megawatt Superphenix fast reactor at Creys Malville, south of Lyons and some 70 km (44 miles) from Geneva.

Although all fast breeders in use or under construction have sodium as coolant and a mixture of plutonium and uranium oxide as fuel, clad in stainless steel, there are two basic versions. One, called the loop design, has sodium flowing through the reactor core and out to a heat exchanger before being pumped back in again. The other, favoured by both Britain and France, is the pool design in which the core sits in a pool of hot liquid sodium while an intermediary circuit of sodium enclosed in piping is pumped through the core to pick up the heat and transfer it to a water circuit by means of a heat exchanger.

The particular advantage of the pool design is that the huge volume of sodium in the core acts as a large heat sink should there be a breakdown in the sodium pumps. Furthermore the secondary sodium circuit can be isolated from the sodium pool should a boiler tube burst and water interact with sodium to generate hydrogen. All fast reactors are now designed with hydrogen flare-off devices in case of accidents in the heat exchangers.

Commercial Electricity Generating Nuclear Reactors in the United States and Canada. The eastern seabord and midwest of the United States has some of the heaviest concentration of nuclear reactors in the world. Nonetheless, no new nuclear reactors have been ordered in the United States since 1978. Canada's reactors are all of the CANDU type.

Commercial Electricity Generating Nuclear Reactors in East and West Europe (see over). The highest concentration of reactors is in France, Belgium and West Germany. France and Belgium both have well over half their electricity generated by nuclear power. The position of Chernobyl can be seen in relation to the rest of Europe.

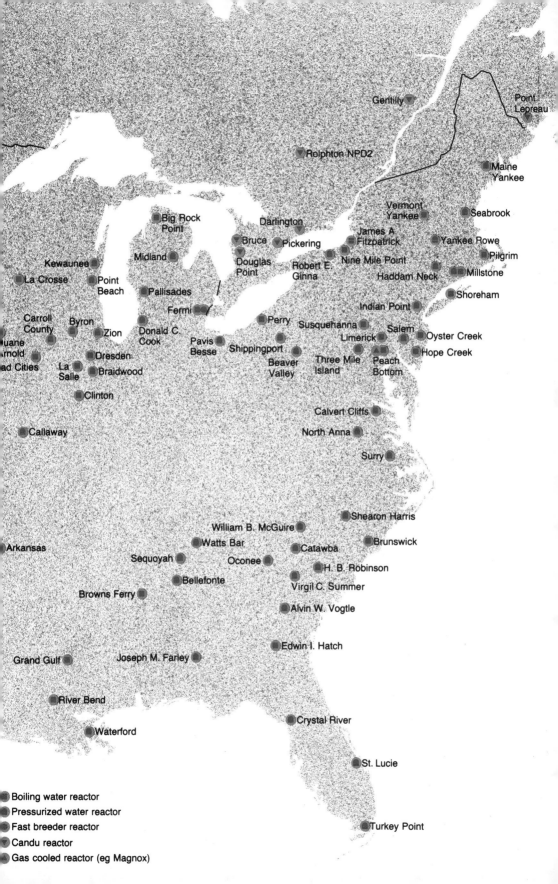

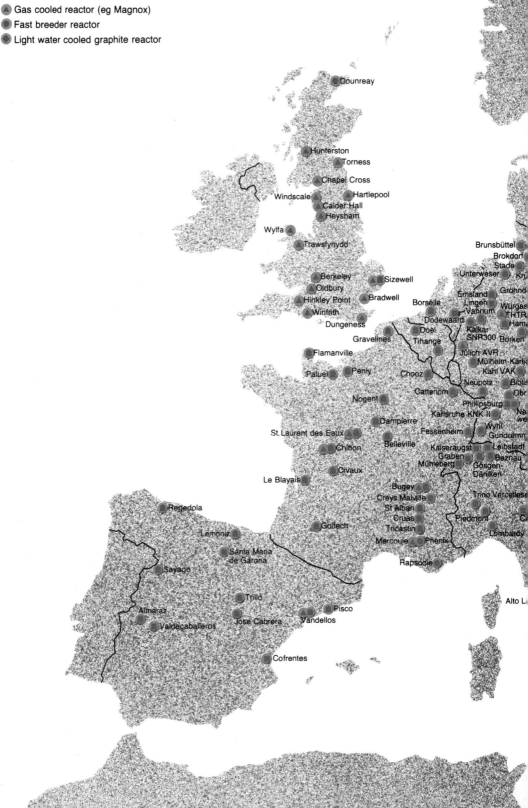

- 🔘 Boiling water reactor
- 🔘 Pressurized water reactor
- 🔺 Gas cooled reactor (eg Magnox)
- 🔘 Fast breeder reactor
- 🔘 Light water cooled graphite reactor

Dounreay

Hunterston
Torness
Chapel Cross
Windscale Hartlepool
Calder Hall
Heysham

Wylfa
Trawsfynydd

Berkeley Sizewell
Oldbury
Hinkley Point Bradwell
Winfrith
Dungeness

Brunsbüttel
Brokdorf
Stade
Unterweser Kr
Emsland Gröhnde
Lingen
Borssele Vahnum Würgas
Dodewaard THTR
Doel Kalkar Ham
Gravelines SNR300 Borken
Tihange
Jülich AVR
Mülheim-Kärli
Kahl VAK
Neupotz Bibli
Ob
Philipsburg
Ne
Karlsruhe KNK II we
Fessenheim Wyhl
Gundremn
Kaiseraugst Leibstadt
Graben Beznau
Mühleberg Gösgen
Däniken

Flamanville
Paluel Penly
Chooz
Cattenom

Nogent

Dampierre

St.Laurent des Eaux
Chinon Belleville

Civaux

Le Blayais

Bugey
Creys Malville
St Alban Trino Vercelles
Cruas
Regedola Tricastin Piedmont
Marcoule Phénix Lombardy
Lemoniz
Golfech
Santa Maria
de Garona Rapsodie

Sayago

Alto L

Trillo
Almaraz Pisco
Jose Cabrera Vandellos
Valdecaballeros

Cofrentes

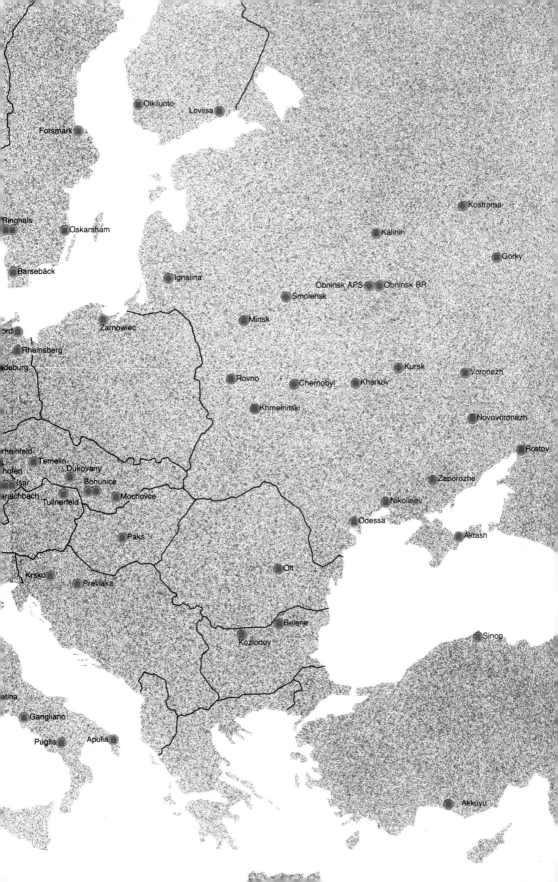

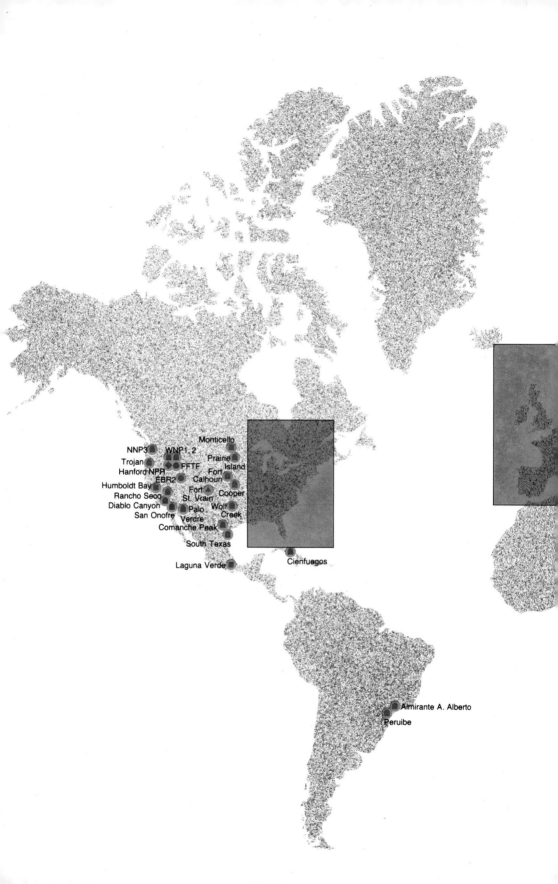

NNP3
WNP1, 2
Monticello
Trojan
Prairie
Hanford NPR
FFTF
Island
EBR2
Fort
Calhoun
Humboldt Bay
Fort
Cooper
Rancho Seco
St. Vrain
Diablo Canyon
Palo
Wolf
San Onofre
Verdre
Creek
Comanche Peak
South Texas
Laguna Verde
Cienfuegos

Almirante A. Alberto
Peruibe

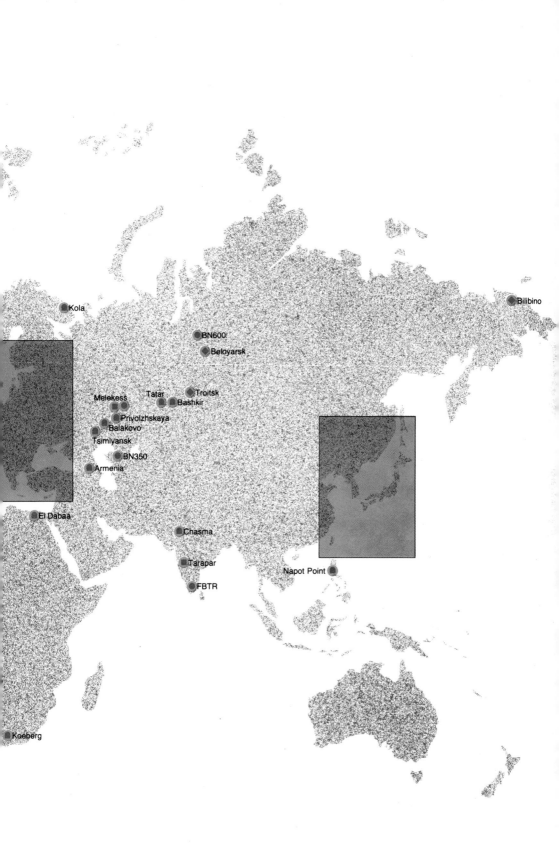

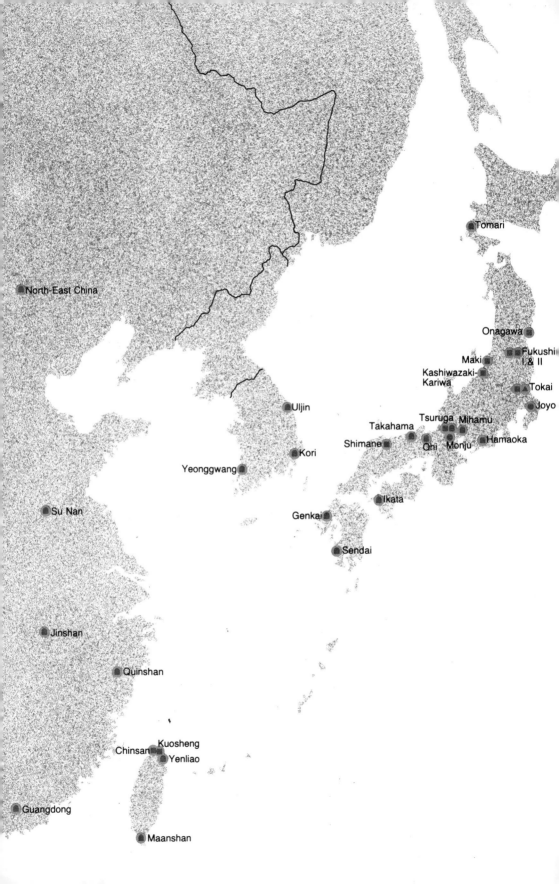

Tomari

North-East China

Onagawa

Maki — Fukushi
I & II

Kashiwazaki-
Kariwa — Tokai

Joyo

Uljin

Tsuruga — Mihamu

Takahama

Shimane — Ohi — Monju — Hamaoka

Kori

Yeonggwang

Su Nan

Ikata

Genkai

Sendai

Jinshan

Quinshan

Kuosheng

Chinsan — Yenliao

Guangdong

Maanshan

The map on the previous page shows the spread of commercial electricity generating nuclear reactors throughout the world except in the boxes drawn out on pages 63, 64-5 and 68. As can be seen, with the exception of the western United States and parts of the Soviet Union, the world has no more than a handful of reactors.

Commercial Electricity Generating Nuclear Reactors in the Far East. Japan in particular has a high proportion of its electricity generated by nuclear power. China has just begun to establish a nuclear power programme with the aid of France and Britain.

The general convention in reactor design is that fuel is placed in the reactor and only withdrawn and replaced after several years of operation. Light water reactors, in particular PWRs, operate at high pressures and after the fuel has been placed in the core, the head of the pressure vessel is bolted on and secured. Approximately once a year the reactor is shut down and the head taken off, so that spent fuel can be removed by remote control and replaced with fresh fuel. Because the fuel does not get consumed evenly throughout the reactor, fuel that has been in the reactor for a short time and still contains useful fissile material is shuffled into a new position. The general idea is to carry out essential maintenance on the reactor while it is shut down for refuelling.

Starting with the Magnox reactors but retaining the concept for the AGRs, British reactor designers set out to achieve refuelling while the reactor was still operating and on load. The refuelling machine can therefore be moved over the top of the head of the reactor, and by remote control remove a plug over the desired fuel channel so that the spent fuel can be hauled out and replaced. From an engineering point of view, the operation is a delicate one because the refuelling machine must lock itself into the channel and maintain the internal gas pressure, and although the system appears to have worked reasonably well for Magnox, it has not proved a great success for AGRs. In fact refuelling of AGRs can be carried out only when the power is down to below 30 per cent of full operating level or excessive vibration is set up in the channel undergoing refuelling.

Reactors that have sets of pressure tubes rather than a single pressure vessel lend themselves to refuelling while still in operation. Both the CANDU and RBMK reactors can therefore be refuelled while on load, and it is tempting to use such systems to extract fuel with good quality plutonium for weapon-making. India, which acquired a CANDU reactor from Canada, did just that to manufacture its first atomic bomb in May 1974.

Reactor operation

The safe operation of a nuclear reactor is a balancing act between no power at all and a runaway chain reaction. There are many different materials in the reactor – steels, uranium fuel, special cladding, moderator, coolant and neutron-absorbing control rods. All of these affect the movement and availability of neutrons, which survive as free particles for only a few thousandths of a second. Moreover, as fuel ages and gets consumed in the reactor, fission products build up, which themselves absorb neutrons and poison the chain reaction. Thus fresh fuel needs more rigorous damping down (by inserting control rods into the spaces between the fuel elements) than aged, nearly spent fuel which, although it still contains fissile material, has become loaded with unwanted fission products.

One important factor in reactor control is temperature, and an increase in temperature enhances the processes governing the rate of fission. For instance, a rise in temperature increases the rate at which uranium-238 absorbs neutrons, with the result that there is a fall in the number of neutrons available for the chain reaction. Therefore, in most of the reactor systems now in use, an unwanted rise in temperature has the fail-safe effect of tending to shut the reactor down.

Each type of reactor behaves in its own, calculable way with regard to reactivity. In a PWR the water in the core has only to get hotter to bring down the reactivity, because of a reduction in water's efficiency as a moderator. Or, if water should escape from the reactor core, then because water doubles up as a moderator and a coolant in a PWR the nuclear reaction is brought to a halt.

As well as acting as moderator, water also absorbs neutrons. So in designing a reactor and trying to make it safe, the physicist must accurately predict which feature is more important in an accident situation. The RBMK, for instance, has a solid graphite moderator, and therefore the neutron-absorbing properties of water are more critical to reactor operation than its moderator capabilities. During the build-up to the Chernobyl explosion, the operators of the RBMK allowed excessive amounts of water in the pressure tubes to flash into steam, and because steam bubbles absorb fewer neutrons than does liquid water, more neutrons suddenly became available. The power therefore began to shoot up. More power means more heat, which automatically means a higher temperature and the formation of more steam. Within seconds the power had risen to a crescendo several hundred times the normal full operating power of the reactor and far beyond any control. Molten, disintegrating fuel interacted violently with water to cause a powerful steam explosion, followed in all probability by a massive hydrogen explosion, the hydrogen having been produced by the interaction of the molten zircalloy cladding with water.

The chain reaction in all reactor systems is kept going through the utilization of two broad categories of neutrons. The great majority of such neutrons – more then 99 per cent – come directly from fissionings and are called 'prompt' neutrons. The remaining 0.5 per cent are known as 'delayed' neutrons and they consist of ones released over varying times from some of the fission products. But whereas the prompt neutrons move from one fissioning to the next in the chain reaction within thousandths of a second at most, and in millionths of a second in fast reactors, the delayed neutrons may take several seconds to appear on the scene.

It is absolutely essential in operating a reactor that a steady chain reaction at the power level desired is sustained through both categories of neutrons, because the delayed fraction provides time for mechanical control rod systems to come into play. If the reactor were kept going on prompt neutrons alone, then insufficient time would be available for the reactor to respond safely. At Chernobyl, the population of neutrons built up until the reactor was prompt critical.

Fast reactors are unique in that the reactivity increases when the fuel compacts. In fact, compaction of the fuel in a fast reactor can lead to small atomic-bomb size explosions, especially if for some reason one chunk of molten fuel gets blasted into another. Meanwhile, nuclear physicists are concerned that should water get into Graphite Moderated Reactors as a result of a burst boiler tube, there is a serious possibility of a Chernobyl-like accident, as the water is driven out of the core by the heat of a nuclear chain reaction.

The spent fuel
At the moment of shut-down of a reactor, the decay heat from the fission products is equivalent in a PWR to some 7 per cent of full power. That may not seem a great amount, but it is sufficient if the heat is not satisfactorily taken away to make the reactor resemble a large 60-tonne steel-melting

furnace, at least for the following 24 hours. The build-up of heat from radioactive decay is rapid. Thus, before a reactor is started up, the amount of radioactive decay from the uranium in the fuel is insufficient even to make the reactor warm. However, within half an hour of the reactor operating at full power, the decay heat reaches three-quarters of its full strength, and after six hours it is up to 90 per cent.

It was the decay heat combined with a lack of cooling that led very nearly to catastrophe at the Three Mile Island PWR plant in 1979. In fact, not all the cooling was lost during the accident, and only part of the reactor core was left clear of water and exposed. Nevertheless, as recent investigations into the reactor pressure vessel have shown, seven years and more after the accident, the temperature reached must have been at least 1,000°C higher where the fuel was exposed than previously estimated. Should all the coolant be lost during reactor operation and it prove impossible to get back-up emergency cooling working in time, the meltdown of the core fuel – even though the actual chain reaction has ceased – would be sufficient to cause the reactor pressure vessel to give way. Enormous quantities of radioactive debris could then escape through the pressure vessel, through the concrete containment base and into the environment, burning their way into the ground. That disastrous scenario has been called the 'China Syndrome' because China lies on the other side of the Earth from the United States where the term was coined.

Nuclear waste

At every stage of the nuclear fuel cycle radioactive waste is generated. After mining, the uranium is enriched and made into fuel rods which then become intensely radioactive after use in the reactor core.

The same fission products that can cause meltdown in a reactor are responsible for many of the problems associated with nuclear waste. One year's operation of a 1-gigawatt reactor (1 gigawatt equals 1,000 million watts) generates some 5 billion curies in the fuel. This represents 70 million times more radioactivity than was originally in the fuel before reactor start-up.

Many of these products are extremely short-lived, hence the intensity of the heat emitted shortly after shut-down. Thus the 180 million curies in each tonne of fuel of a PWR at shut-down (after operating at full power) drops 260 times to 693,000 curies after a year, and to just 470 curies after

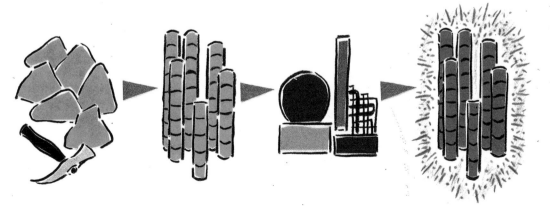

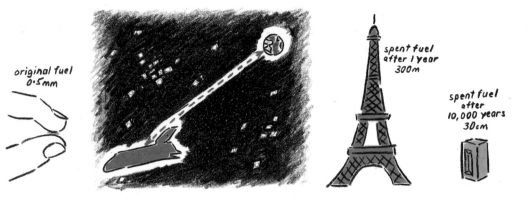

original fuel
0·5mm

spent fuel
after 1 year
300m

spent fuel
after
10,000 years
30cm

10,000 years. But even 470 is a dangerous quantity, and so radioactive waste must be kept isolated from human beings and the environment for a very long time indeed.

Three broad categories of radioactive substances are generated in a reactor: fission products, transuranics and activation products. Yet the bulk of the spent fuel consists of unused uranium. Ideally the operator would like more uranium-235 to be consumed before the reactor needed refuelling, but the build-up of fission products – especially some that poison the chain reaction – makes it impractical. The hundred or so fission products also account for most of the radioactivity in the spent fuel. Some of these vanish (by decay) very quickly; others, such as caesium-137 and strontium-90, have half-lives in the region of 30 years.

The part of the nuclear waste in spent fuel called transuranics, or actinides, are elements that are heavier in mass than the uranium from which they have been derived. Plutonium is a transuranic, as is americium-241, which is derived from plutonium-241 by beta decay (but is itself an alpha-emitter). The transuranics make up no more than 3 per cent of the total radioactivity in fuel that has cooled for six months but as the short-life decays the transuranic becomes relatively more important.

Another group of important radioactive substances formed in a working nuclear reactor are the activation products. These are created through neutron bombardment of both structural and active components of reactors, such as moderators, coolants and steel structures. Activation products such as tritium (an isotope of hydrogen) formed in the cooling water of light water reactors or carbon-14 in the carbon dioxide coolant of gas cooled reactors tend to be discharged into the environment during the normal operation of the plant, often in considerable quantities. Activation products in the structural components take on particular relevance when it comes to repairing and maintaining the reactor, or at the end of the reactor's life when it is finally decommissioned and ultimately dismantled.

Even when a modern PWR is operating normally and to specification, it releases into the environment radioactive substances that contribute to the gradual build-up of background radiation. Each year a PWR routinely discharges into the air some 54 curies of krypton-85, 6-8 curies of krypton-88, 620 curies of xenon-133, 8 curies of carbon-14 and an unspecified amount of long-lived radio-iodine. The total atmospheric dose from one reactor each year amounts to some 40 person-sieverts. This dose is delivered

Radioactivity builds up enormously in a nuclear reactor. Thus, compared to the very low level of radio activity in the fresh fuel, spent fuel is 200 million times more radioactive when first taken from the reactor as if 100 kilometres out in space compared to the original amount represented as 0.5 mm held between the fingers. The radioactivity quickly decays away, falling 300 times over the first year. Nevertheless after 10,000 years the spent fuel is still 600 times more radioactive than it was originally in the fresh fuel.

to the body over the time required for the radioactive isotopes to decay away.

Tritium is also released into both the atmosphere and into water. Whereas a Magnox releases an average of some 36 curies per year, a PWR can be expected to release 30 curies into the air each year and 1,550 curies into water.

All these radionuclides, even the inert gas krypton, have biological effects on the body. Krypton-85, for instance, has a physical half-life of 10.7 years and emits both beta and gamma particles. It is extremely soluble in human fat and therefore tends to find its way into all parts of the body. Nevertheless, it gives the greatest dose to the lungs and blood-forming tissues. Krypton-85 also gets into animal fat, so adding to the human dose if the animals are eaten. Furthermore, because of krypton's predeliction for fat, women (especially pregnant women) are likely to be more at risk from krypton-85 than are men.

Carbon-14, with its 5,700-year half-life, is both a fission product and an activation product brought about through neutron interactions with carbon, nitrogen and oxygen. Because carbon is a component of all organic molecules in living organisms, it finds its way into humans. A 1,000-megawatt PWR generates some 12 curies each year in the primaray coolant circuit. Some 4 curies per year get discharged with water into the environment, and 8 curies into the air.

Some scientists estimate that the worldwide dose from just one PWR is likely to cause between 80 and 240 cancer deaths each year just from the releases into the atmosphere. Research on radiation workers who had been contaminated with tritium indicates that it takes several years to eliminate from the body. Tritium, being a form of hydrogen, finds its way into genetic material, where it is bound tightly, thus causing genetic effects and abnormal development. The routine discharge of more than 1,000 curies of tritium each year from light water reactors must inevitably cause harm to health, although the extent of such effects will depend on how much tritium gets caught up in the food chain and into human beings.

Cobalt-60 is also discharged in small quantities from nuclear reactors. The danger for humans results from the cobalt becoming incorporated into vitamin B_{12} (cyanocobalamin). In that form it is readily taken into the body and retained.

Worker exposure

In their work at nuclear power plants, people concerned with operation and maintenance inevitably receive external radiation, for the most part from gamma radiation. They may also receive elevated internal doses from radionuclides routinely discharged into the air and water. The United Nations Scientific Committee on the Effects of Atomic Radiation (UNSCEAR) estimated that on average each megawatt of electricty generated at nuclear power stations gives a yearly dose to the occupationally exposed worker of 10 millisieverts.

One might have expected the radiation dose to workers, as well as to the general public, to fall as experience is gained with nuclear power. However findings in the United States suggest that the opposite is happening. Thus while the electricity generated by nuclear power plants increased some 23 times between 1969 and 1979, from 1,300 megawatts to 30,000 megawatts, worker exposure increased 32 times over that same period, from 12.47 person-sieverts in 1969 to 397.59 person-sieverts in 1979. At the same time the number of workers required for each megawatt of electricty generated increased by more than 3 times. One reason was the additional number of workers required to carry out repairs on aging plants, combined with the requirement to limit total exposure to any one individual.

Decommissioning and activation products
The nuclear industry believed until the late 1970s that most of the radioactivity induced in the structure of a reactor, therefore in the pressure vessel, piping and heat exchangers, was short-lived. Thus the first stage in decommissioning a reactor at the end of its life would be to take out all the fuel, then to encase the entire structure in concrete to prevent any access, and finally in the last stage to dismantle it and bury the pieces, either in a repository on land or in the bottom of the ocean. The site would therefore be returned to something of its original state, and if needed another reactor could be built at the same location.

However, in 1976 physicists in the United States discovered that radioactive nickel-59 would be formed in significant amounts during the 30-year lifetime of the plant, and here the problem is the long half-life, some 80,000 years. Thus after 100 years the activity will have been reduced by no more than a small fraction of the total. Worse was to come with the discovery of an even more powerful gamma-emitter, also with a long half-life. This is niobium-94. In 1981 the US Nuclear Regulatory Comission indicated that the dose rate from niobium-94 would be some 170 grays per year with an additional 8 grays coming from the radioactive nickel. A person standing or working close to such a source of radiation for any length of time would therefore soon exceed the maximum permissible level, even at the higher levels allowed for workers in the nuclear industry. As a result, robotics are increasingly being used for maintenance and repair.

Various attempts are now being made to dismantle derelict reactors. Most of these are prototypes and therefore relatively small. Nevertheless the process of dismantling them is proving to be time-consuming and costly.

One of the first reactors to be dismantled was the small Elk River reactor in the United States, which operated for only a short time before it was shut down. During dismantling it was discovered that an unprotected worker standing next to the core support plate at the bottom of the pressure vessel would receive his maximum permissible 3-monthly radiation dose in less than a couple of seconds. The 15 men involved in cutting the steel reactor vessel into pieces had therefore to work under water, using remotely operated plasma cutting torches. The metal fragments from the reactor contained some 370 million million becquerels of radioactivity and totalled some 600 tonnes of dangerous scrap metal. Nearly 3,000 cubic metres of contaminated concrete also had to be shipped away from the site and buried in a special repository.

The United States has now embarked on dismantling the somewhat larger Shippingport reactor, which began operation in 1958 and continued through the 1970s. The cutting up will take at least five years and give rise to 11,700 cubic metres of radioactive waste – almost as much as is being produced in the clean-up of the Three Mile Island Number 2 reactor. The waste is to go to the military site at Hanford in Washington State. A larger

Several different kinds of radioactive waste are produced in a nuclear power station. Some are discharged routinely during operation from the reactor, others are discharged when the spent fuel is taken from the reactor and some are generated in the construction materials by neutron bombardment.

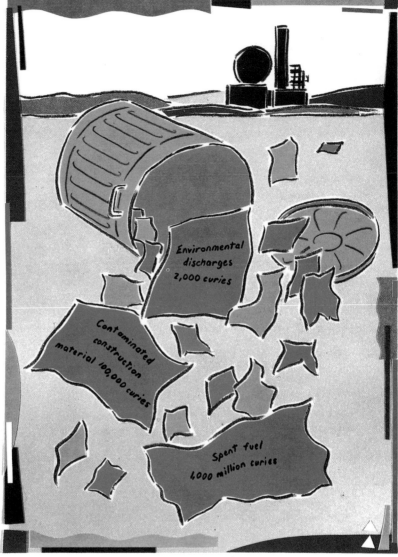

Environmental discharges 2,000 curies

Contaminated construction material 100,000 curies

Spent fuel 4,000 million curies

reactor in the the one-gigawatt range will generate some 8,000 cubic metres of contaminated steel and concrete.

One idea currently being discussed is to avoid cutting up the pressure vessel. Instead the concrete containment would be broken open and the pressure vessel, after detaching it from its ducts and other restraints, would be lifted out, covered in concrete to cut down gamma radiation and dropped somewhere in the ocean. Such a method of disposal has not received international approval.

But the really vexed problems of dismantling come when there have been accidents, as at Three Mile Island and at Chernobyl. In both those reactors, the fuel has crumbled and is no longer in a state that it can be removed easily.

At Chernobyl the reactor ruin has been smothered in concrete. For the time being that concrete coating is keeping radioactive levels in the vicinity of the original reactor sufficiently low for operators to start up the neighbouring Number 3 reactor. But how long will the encasement last? Undoubtedly the concrete will begin deteriorating after a few years, and the problem then will be to ensure that the contained radioactivity does not start leaking out. Chernobyl is likely to remain a smouldering problem for many hundreds of years.

Reprocessing

The plutonium generated in a reactor is embedded in a matrix of the original fuel. It is therefore surrounded by uranium atoms as well as a host of virulently radioactive fission products. The plutonium has therefore to be extracted from the fuel, and the process used to do this is a chemical one – called reprocessing. In fact, the spent fuel is dissolved in nitric acid and uranium and transuranics such as plutonium separated out from the bulk of the fission products using special organic solvents. By mixing the phosphate-based oil solvent with a water-based solvent, the plutonium separates out from the uranium and can be converted to an extractable solid after oxidation. When the original fuel for the reactor has been enriched with uranium-235, then the uranium in spent fuel will contain more useful uranium-235 than is present in natural uranium. It too, like the plutonium, offers potential energy if recycled through a reactor. Reprocessing was originally devised for the extraction of plutonium for military purposes. But it then came to be seen as an essential step in maximizing the use of nuclear reactors for power generation. Indeed, a fast reactor that breeds relatively large quantities of plutonium must be linked to a reprocessing facility to make the plutonium available for fuel.

Today, there is a considerable debate over the future of reprocessing, and it hinges on several issues. For one, reprocessing turns a solid fuel with most of the fission products held within it into an intensely radioactive liquid. That liquid has then to be kept in special long-lasting, actively cooled stainless steel tanks until such time as it can be solidified. Reprocessing is controversial because of the radioactive wastes that inevitably get released into the environment, discharged into the atmosphere and into waterways.

The importance of fast reactors and plutonium to the future of nuclear power depends intrinsically on the quantities of uranium in the Earth's crust and how readily it can be mined. Uranium deposits are fairly widespread, and the issue is not the total amount (probably about a million million tonnes) but its concentration. In fact, a uranium content of less than 50 parts per million of other minerals gives no more energy in a light water reactor than would coal in a coal-fired power station for the amount of ore that would have to be mined. And because the cost of building a nuclear power station is so much higher than that of constructing a conventional fossil-fuel station, such ore cannot be considered to be economic (at least until the supply of oil and coal runs out).

Even with uranium deposits that can be mined economically, the amounts of overburden and rock that have to be removed are vast. For

In reprocessing, nitric acid is used to dissolve the uranium fuel so that the plutonium and unused uranium can be extracted. The rest, including fission products, is nuclear waste and has to be disposed of safely.

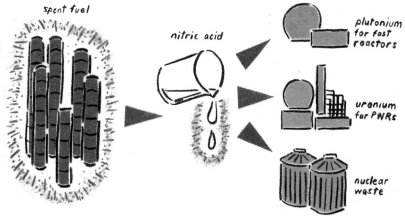

spent fuel

nitric acid

plutonium for fast reactors

uranium for PWRs

nuclear waste

instance, open-pit mining in the Colorado Plateau leads to 2 million tonnes of overburden being shifted to extract 85,700 tonnes of carnotite ore that will provide a 1-gigawatt reactor with enough fuel for one year. In fact, 6.5 hectares (16 acres) of land have to be dug open for each gigawatt of electricty generated in a year, and the abandoned tailings put the environment at risk for thousands of years to come.

The enormous quantities of energy residing in an atom of uranium have therefore given the illusion of it being almost a miracle fuel. In fact, the finished fuel pellet is the product of a long, complicated extraction and fuel fabrication process, with vast amounts of overburden, rock and tailings (as well as depleted uranium from the uranium enrichment plant) being cast on one side.

Estimates of the total reserves of uranium that would be available from ore of sufficient quality to make it economically worthwhile to mine vary from 4 million to 10 million tonnes. Consumed in thermal reactors, such an amount would provide 500 1-gigawatt plants with enough uranium for no more than 60 to 100 years. In 1979, the European Centre for Nuclear Research (CERN) in Geneva came up with the forecast that the energy obtainable from the total world recoverable reserves of uranium, if burned in thermal reactors like the PWR, would amount to no more than one-fifth of the energy still remaining in recoverable reserves of petroleum and in strict economic terms at least five times more expensive.

Fast reactors cost twice as much to build as do PWRs, and they depend absolutely on being fuelled with plutonium derived from thermal reactors. They therefore depend on reprocessing. But reprocessing has proved increasingly expensive, particularly as more stringent requirements are placed on the levels of discharges that can legitimately be permitted.

To sustain a reasonable-sized programme of fast reactors requires that the plutonium in spent fuel be extracted as soon as possible, otherwise the supply of fresh plutonium will lag behind the demand. And if too large a programme of thermal reactors is used, the opportunities of breeding plutonium in the future will fade as uranium-235 is consumed. Yet, the gamma radiation from fast-reactor fuel which has cooled for just 5 months is 50 times greater than from PWR fuel that has cooled for 5 years. The

77

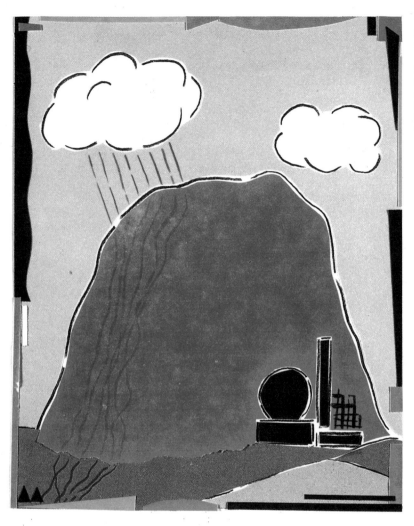

The fuel for running a nuclear reactor for one year comes from some 100,000 tons of rock, most of which gets left as tailings on the ground, causing radioactive contamination of the environment.

economic penalties in devising a method for reprocessing such very active material and for properly protecting the workforce and public are high.

Another possibility is to recycle plutonium and unused uranium-235 in thermal reactor systems. In theory, the plutonium and uranium derived in that way would give an extra 40 per cent of energy on top of that in the original thermal fuel. But the recycled uranium is contaminated with neutron-absorbing uranium-236 and uranium-234, both of which drastically reduce the value of the recycled uranium as fissile material.

Meanwhile the presence of uranium-232 causes radiological problems during enrichment, fabrication and fuel-handling. Indeed, three years after its initial discharge from the reactor, gamma emissions from uranium-232 will make recycled fuel 20 times more radioactive than fuel fabricated from fresh uranium.

The use of plutonium in thermal reactors is also problematical. Plutonium-241 decays into americium-241, so that within 14 years of discharge from the reactor some 6 per cent of potentially fissile material is lost. Meanwhile, both plutonium-240 and plutonium-242 are neutron absorbers, and because these isotopes together comprise nearly 30 per cent of the plutonium derived from PWRs, their presence makes a significant difference to the fissile value of recycled plutonium. Consequently the number of times such plutonium can be recycled is severely limited.

Reprocessing plants

At present opinion is divided about whether reprocessing should be carried out at all. Several nuclear physicists and engineers are critical of fast-reactor programmes, believing that any benefits they offer do not justify the costs and risks. This criticism includes reprocessing plants because they are an essential component of a fast-reactor fuel cycle.

Attempts to operate plants for reprocessing spent fuels from commercial reactors have generally run into difficulties. In New York State, Nuclear Fuel Services operated a reprocessing plant for seven years between 1966 and 1973, by which time it achieved a total throughput of only 600 tonnes – barely 30 per cent of its intended performance.

Now, with the plant shut down, New York State has 600,000 gallons of high-level waste to deal with, costing several million dollars a year in maintenance, and a potential bill of more than 1,000 million dollars – 30 times the original cost – to decommission the plant.

France, meanwhile, has built reprocessing plants at Cap de la Hague in Normandy and at Marcoule in the south. With its large PWR programme, the country is setting out to reprocess spent PWR fuel at la Hague, having adapted the original plant from its use merely for spent Magnox fuel – which is now sent to Marcoule for reprocessing. Britain has also set out to reprocess spent thermal oxide fuel, in a plant under construction known as THORP – Thermal Oxide Reprocessing Plant – for which planning permission was received after a 6-month-long public inquiry in 1977. As with France, the Japanese have been looked to for financial help.

Sellafield, and its operator British Nuclear Fuels, have been under a barrage of criticism over the past ten years for shoddy operating procedures and for a high level of discharge into the environment. Invidious comparisons have been made between Sellafield and other reprocessing plants, in particular with Cap de la Hague.

Currently at Sellafield only Magnox fuel is reprocessed, the attempt at reprocessing higher burn-up thermal oxide fuel having ended in a disastrous accident in which 35 workers were contaminated with the beta-emitter ruthenium-106, which blew out of the process line. Reprocessing actually increases the volume of wastes by as much as 100 times or more by liquefying the spent fuel. The increase in volume after reprocessing Magnox fuel is some 160 times, although the intensely radioactive part of the waste is reduced in volume by one-third. Meanwhile all the krypton-85 and tritium originally in the spent fuel are discharged into the atmosphere, along with some carbon-14.

When spent fuel is extracted from a reactor core, it must be allowed to cool down safely and the usual practice is to put it in a special water-filled cooling pond near the reactor. In the United States, because of the moratorium on commercial reprocessing, all spent fuel is now kept on site. The ponds, although limited in size, are being adapted to take a number of years' spent fuel by compacting it and altering the stacking arrangements. Considerable quantities of heat are generated by all the stacks of fuel, and the integrity of the pond and its cooling system must be maintained for the time that the fuel remains in it. The total inventory of radioactive substances in the fuel is extremely large, enough to melt the fuel should cooling cease for any length of time. Therefore in any one reactor site the quantities of radioactive waste amount to many thousands of times the fall-out from one atomic bomb.

In countries such as Britain and France, which have their own reprocessing facilities, the spent fuel is first stored at the reactor site in the station cooling pond. It is then fitted into massive steel flasks and transported by rail and road to the reprocessing plant, where it is again put in a cooling pond to await treatment. Some concern has been expressed over the safety of the flasks should there be an accident in transit, especially a collision followed by an intense chemical fire (such as from an overturned petrol tanker). The operators have deliberately subjected flasks to collisions and to fires, and say that they are able to withstand foreseeable accidents.

Fast-reactor spent fuel, on the other hand, comes into a category of its own because of its high heat output. Indeed, an irradiated fuel assembly from a fast reactor may generate as much as 30 killowatts of heat – far too much for a conventional cooling pond – and sodium-filled containers have to be used. At present, fast-reactor fuel is sent from Malville in the south of France all the way to the United Kingdom Atomic Energy Authority's fast reactor site at Dounreay in Scotland.

During the 1970s, hold-ups in the reprocessing of spent Magnox fuel at Sellafield led to an unexpected problem of corrosion of the stored fuel in the cooling pond. The Magnox cladding became pitted, and water came into contact with the spent fuel, with the result that some of the more soluble radionuclides (such as caesium) began to escape in considerable quantities. The result was that in the mid-1970s the discharges of caesium-137 alone amounted to some 120,000 curies a year.

In fact, between 1977 and 1980 Sellafield's annual discharges of beta-emitters such as caesium-137 and plutonium-241 were seven times worse than from La Hague. Over the same period Sellafield discharged 200 times more alpha-emitters (such as plutonium and americium) into the sea.

In recent years British Nuclear Fuels has embarked on a major investment programme to improve its discharges. BNFL has thus reduced beta discharges to less than one-tenth of the peak levels of the mid-1970s. An Enhanced Actinide Removal Plant (EARP) is to be commissioned in the early 1990s, the ultimate aim being to bring down the levels of alpha discharges to those achieved at la Hague.

The operation and maintenance of reprocessing plants leads to considerable worker exposure to both external and internal radiation. Reprocessing can therefore be seen as an intrinsically awkward and polluting part of the nuclear fuel cycle, and one that gives considerable external exposures to the workforce as well as to the general public in the vicinity of the plant. Indeed, consumer behaviour with regard to the eating of fish and shellfish has altered perceptibly as the public has come to recognize the extent to which their local environment has been contaminated. Waters off the coast of north-western England now show concentrations of plutonium and americium that are some 2,000 times higher than fall-out levels, while even

80

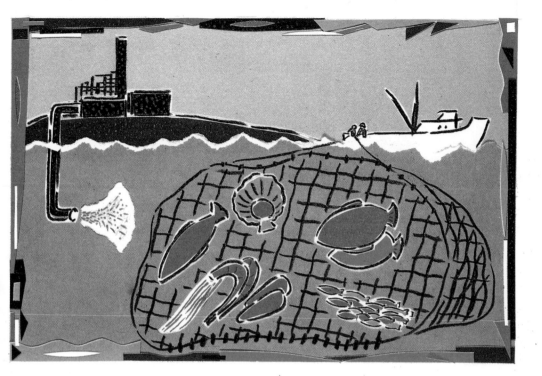

Routine, as well as accidental, discharges from a nuclear installation lead to varying degrees of radioactive contamination of sea-food.

the North Sea has double the fall-out levels because of Sellafield discharges. Sellafield has been plagued by accidents, many of them serious. Various installations on the site have leaked – some for years before being detected and only after many thousands of curies had run off into the soil. For instance, a silo containing the cladding from spent Magnox fuel leaked for at least four years before the leak was discovered, by which time as much as 50,000 curies (most of it caesium) had escaped. Another leak from a building containing high-level waste was discovered in 1978, by which time as much as 100,000 curies had probably escaped. During 1985, half a tonne of reprocessed uranium was discharged into the Irish Sea, an accident that had much in common with the accidental discharge of solvent and radioactive crud containing at least 4,500 curies of waste in November 1983. Also in 1986 some 15 reprocessing workers became internally contaminated with plutonium nitrate after it had escaped through a faulty valve. Several workers received well above the maximum permissible levels for plutonium exposure.

The West German authorities have persistently tried to build a reprocessing plant. But so far all attempts have been foiled by vigorous opposition from environmentalists. The first major effort was to establish a plant at Gorleben, a village close to the East German border in the state of Niedersachsen. But the furore it aroused among the public was such that in May 1979 both the Federal government and the government of Lower Saxony had to abandon their plans.

However, West Germany has been trying again, this time in Lower Bavaria at Wackersdorf, close to the Austrian border. Even before Chernobyl, the project aroused enormous antagonism on both sides of the border, and the question remains whether the project will proceed or like its predecessor have to be abandoned.

Japan had a reprocessing plant built for it by French engineers at Tokai Mura, which first came into operation some ten years ago. The installation has hardly been a success, between 1978 and 1985 averaging no more than 14 per cent of its intended capacity of 200 tonnes of spent fuel a year. Particular problems were found with high burn-up spent fuel from PWRs, which caused corrosion and pitting of the dissolvers, so that they had to be replaced after five years instead of lasting for ten as designed. Discharges into the environment have also been high, with krypton-85 being released untrapped. The plant has also failed to control its discharges of iodine-129, and in one year alone (1985) discharged more than 7,000 curies of tritium. After treating a total of 253 tonnes of spent fuel, some 224 cubic metres of high-level waste had accumulated in the storage tank.

The Electricity Utilities of Japan now plan to construct an 800-tonne per year reprocessing plant at Rokkasho-Mura. Meanwhile they have contracted with BNFL in Britain and COGEMA in France for the reprocessing of 5,900 tonnes of spent fuel. The contract allows for the wastes to be returned to Japan in a conditioned form at intervals up to the year 2005.

～～ Waste disposal ～～

The public has become increasingly anxious about what the nuclear industry intends to do with all the accumulating nuclear waste. Various options have been put forward, and they range from dispatching the waste into space on the back of a rocket to dropping it judiciously into the Mid-atlantic Trench and leaving movements of the Earth's crust to take the waste ever deeper. Other choices include drilling bore holes several thousands of metres deep either into rock on land or out at sea, digging out caverns, again either on land or at sea (with a tunnel to the land), or building mausoleum-like structures on the surface of the land.

The industry believes that different kinds of nuclear wastes need different kinds of disposal. The most radioactive obviously needs the greatest care – and the deepest disposal – whereas low-level waste requires little more than sub-surface disposal, not very different from modern methods of landfill.

If spent fuel has been reprocessed, the disposal of waste requires a somewhat different approach than if the fuel has been left intact, as is now the practice in countries such as the United States and to an increasing extent in Sweden. In the United States the consensus both within the nuclear industry and the environmental movement is that the spent fuel should be stored in special self-cooling structures, designed to draw in a natural circulation of air.

Nevertheless, spent fuel is accumulating at a considerable rate, threatening to clog the system before sufficient facilities can be built. More than 20,000 spent fuel assemblies – the product of little more than 20 years of reactor operation – are now stored temporarily in spent fuel ponds throughout the United States, and the number is increasing by some 4,000 each year. By the end of the century the number could be 300,000.

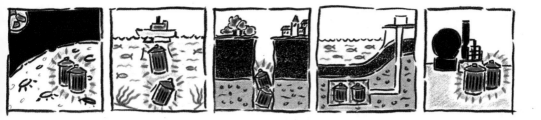

Dumping: various options have been proposed for getting rid of radioactive waste: sending it off into outer space by rocket, depositing it on the sea-bed, dumping it in bore holes, placing it in caverns dug under the sea-bed, or storing it on site at the power station.

For reprocessed fuel, the first concern is to find a satisfactory way of solidifying the high-level waste in storage tanks. Again the problem is acute in the United States, where 30,000 cubic metres of high-level liquid and solid waste are now stored in aging steel tanks. Similarly there are some 2 million cubic metres of low-level wastes, of which 500,000 cubic metres contain transuranic alpha-emitters in shallow burial and already leaching from the disposal site towards groundwater. In fact three out of six shallow dump sites in the United States have been closed because of off-site contamination and breaches in packaging and transport regulations.

In Sweden, low-level and intermediate-level waste is now being stored in a cavern carved out of granite rock off the coast with access from the shore. The repository is therefore under the sea bed, but not at any great depth. The intention, meanwhile, is to bury high-level wastes derived from spent fuel that has been sent to France for reprocessing down shafts at least 500 metres in depth.

West Germany is looking to abandoned salt mines as a repository for its nuclear waste. But the programme has run into some problems because parts of the area being investigated have proved to be less stable geologically than would be required for the long periods of time the wastes have to remain isolated from the environment.

From stories, later backed up by strong evidence, that emerged from the Soviet Union in late 1957, it would appear that nuclear wastes can give rise to massive explosions if not properly attended. The accident occurred in the Urals and led to the evacuation of 30 villages and communities and to a number of radiation victims, although precise numbers have never been revealed. Research in the United States in the late 1970s at the Oak Ridge National Laboratory suggests that the accident may have occurred in a nuclear waste storage facility following the failure of a cooling system in a high-level waste storage tank. According to a nuclear physicist, Lev Tumerman, who later emigrated to Israel and who had driven through the stricken area in 1960, signposts commanded drivers to drive through at maximum speed and not stop for 30 kilometres (19 miles). 'On both sides of the road, as far as I could see, the land was dead; no towns, only chimneys of destroyed houses, no cultivated fields or pastures, no herds, no people . . . nothing', he observed.

CHAPTER

4

Nuclear accidents

Already the nuclear industry, in its relatively brief history, has had serious accidents which have led to the release of large quantities of radioactive materials into the environment. Two occurred within weeks of each other: the fire in the Number 1 pile in the British reactor at Windscale, brought about when the graphite moderator overheated, and the disaster in the Soviet reactor at Kyshtym in the Urals.

In the 1957 accident at Windscale, scientists in charge of the plutonium pile were trying to release pent-up energy. The method of releasing it involves heating the graphite beyond its normal operating temperature, and on that occasion it all went wrong. By the time the fire raging in the core had been put out, some 20,000 curies of iodine-131 had escaped into the surrounding countryside, and the resulting radioactive plume swept across Britain to Denmark and over the European continent. Part of it also passed across the Irish Sea to Ireland.

Fall-out from the plume was washed out during its passage, but undoubtedly the greatest contamination occurred close to the reactor itself. And although the British government initially underplayed the full nature of the accident, within days bans on the sale of milk from farms in the locality went into force. Hundreds of thousands of gallons of milk had to be poured away because it contained high levels of iodine-131.

Despite such precautions, the cancer toll as the result of the accident may top 1,000. But this number is barely discernible given that the normal rate of cancer in the population is one out of four for women and one out of five for men (taking all causes of death into account).

Every attempt was made to cover up the implications of the Windscale fire of 1957. No advice was given to the public in the vicinity or indeed in the path of the plume to take simple precautions – such as staying indoors when the radiation in the air had reached its peak.

Chernobyl was a wholly different story. In 1957 Britain was the only European country west of the Soviet Union to have nuclear power stations, and very few of its neighbours had the resources to measure radioactive fall-out except in the most hit-and-miss way. By the time of Chernobyl in 1986, all European countries had networks of radiation-monitoring stations, particularly in sensitive areas such as those close to nuclear power plants.

It was therefore no coincidence that the first indication in the West of a nuclear disaster somewhere in the Soviet Union, and very quickly pinned down to the Ukraine, was from abnormally high readings of radioactivity in the air at the Forsmark nuclear power station on the eastern side of Sweden. Indeed, when workers arrived at the Swedish station on the morning of 28

April 1986, they were stopped from entering the plant because of contamination on their faces, hands and clothing. Activity was also found on cars in the car park, on the ground, and in puddles of water. Routine precautions were then taken as if the radioactivity were escaping from the Forsmark set of boiling water reactors. Workers were therefore sent away and both local and central authorities were notified to put them in a state of readiness for carrying out routine emergency action and establishing countermeasures.

Within an hour of the notification, an emergency organization was already set up at the Swedish National Institute of Radiation Protection, growing in numbers to some 100 people and remaining active for 24 hours a day over the first months following the accident at Chernobyl. Within the first day, the emergency task force had concluded that evacuation of any of the Swedish population, sheltering them or advising them to take iodine tablets to counter fall-out of radioactive iodine would not be justified. Similar conclusions were reached throughout western Europe, although more careful analysis of the situation in hot-spot areas revealed later that a more judicious approach might well have been followed.

One of the first reactions of the nuclear establishment in the West was to dissociate its own nuclear industry from that in the Soviet Union. Accusations – such as that the Chernobyl reactor lacked adequate containment, or that it was a reactor type that would never have been licensed under Western conditions – were rife. But, as details emerged and more knowledgeable scientists made themselves heard, it had later to be admitted

In the 'China Syndrome' red-hot molten fuel eats its way through the reactor pressure vessel and bursts through the concrete containment into the soil and groundwater.

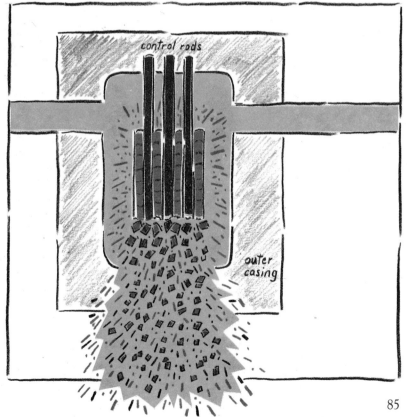

that the Chernobyl RBMK had a containment as good as many containment structures in the West. It used basically the same principles of preventing a pressure build up through a steam-suppression system. In Britain, for example, the majority of reactors – the Magnox type – have no more than a flimsy structure, designed more to keep operational doses down than to withstand explosions.

The next phase was a clamp-down of explicit information in the West on the extent of fall-out. The classic example occurred in France where the man responsible for nuclear safety, Professor Pellerin, actually denied that the plume had crossed into France; it was supposed to have made a detour along the border with West Germany, but keeping always on the German side. Only later, through private initiatives, did it emerge that some parts of France had been badly contaminated, in particular the Drome region and Corsica.

Indeed, the nuclear industry in the West suddenly saw itself threatened by the Soviet accident, for if it could happen there could it not also happen in a Western reactor? Public confidence in the nuclear industry was faltering. Opinion polls throughout the world showed a strong shift of feeling from acceptability to mistrust. Today, the nuclear industry feels it can ride out the storm. In terms of immediate deaths, hardly more people died after Chernobyl than died in the fire at London's King's Cross underground station in November 1987. Some nuclear proponents believe that the Chernobyl accident may prove to be a blessing in disguise for nuclear power. The worst had happened and the public could see that the world had not been decimated. Yet such attitudes did not take into account the thousands of people who would contract cancer or pass on genetic defects to their children, as a result of Chernobyl. They would be the unseen, unnoticed victims of the disaster.

The Chernobyl accident showed that places as far away as 2,000 kilometres (1,250 miles) from the site could be affected. It also showed graphically that the 2-kilometre (1-mile) evacuation zone around a nuclear station planned for in Britain in the event of a major radiation release was grossly inadequate. The problem in western Europe is made worse by high population density. Compared with the Soviet Union, many more people live relatively close to nuclear plants in countries such as Britain, Belgium, West Germany and parts of France. If, for instance, an accident of the magnitude of Chernobyl had happened at one of the two Biblis plants on the Rhine River near Mannheim in West Germany, a 30-kilometre (19-mile) evacuation zone would take in 2.3 million people, compared with the 100,000 around Chernobyl. Moreover, just 50 kilometres (31 miles) away from the Biblis nuclear station are Wiesbaden and Frankfurt, each with an additional 2.7 million people. The Indian Point plant near New York City has some 1.5 million people in its 30- kilometre range.

Modern nuclear reactors such as those at Chernobyl contain enormous quantities of radioactive waste, up to a thousand times the amount released in one Hiroshima-sized explosion. Just ten per cent of the core inventory of radionuclides escaping into the environment is still a hundred times a Hiroshima bomb. That fact would explain why certain areas such as Neuherberg, close to Munich, received radioactive iodine and caesium over a two-day period – April 29 to 30 – at levels between 50 and 100 times those observed during the atmospheric bomb testing peak of the 1960s.

Starting in the Ukraine, the Chernobyl plume first travelled northwards over east Europe and Scandinavia and then spread westwards over West Germany, France, Italy, The Netherlands, Switzerland and across the English Channel over Britain. Another segment of the plume passed over Yugoslavia and spread over Turkey and Greece. Fall-out was particularly heavy in certain regions because of rain washing through the plume.

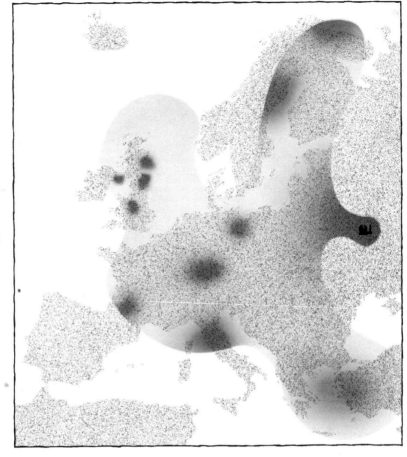

Most radiation authorities were caught by surprise at the way certain places, 1,500 kilometres (nearly 1,000 miles) away from the stricken reactor, could suddenly get doused and receive many times more fall-out than a place nextdoor. Moreover, most calculations derived from hypothetical accidents were based on the premise that a radiation release would take place over a relatively short period of time and not extend over several weeks as did the Chernobyl accident, which involved a secondary peak of release some ten days after the initial explosion. Equally the scientists had not foreseen the extent to which a vast area such as eastern and western Europe could be affected by one accident alone, and the degree to which the contamination remained high in certain hilly areas.

Despite their conviction before Chernobyl that the chances of major radiation releases from nuclear reactors were extremely small, nuclear industry scientists and those who set the safety standards must plan for accidents and determine radiation levels at which different responses are called for. Evacuation is the most extreme response, followed by sheltering, and then by banning or limiting the consumption of certain foodstuffs.

Everything has to be taken into account: the amount we breathe in from the plume, the amount we receive simply from being outside and exposed to

87

gamma radiation, as well as from deposits on our clothes and skin; what kind of house we live in and whether the walls are thick enough to protect us; what we eat and where the produce comes from; how much we wash and shower. Indeed, after a bad accident at a nuclear power plant we have to consider every aspect of our lives to decide whether we need to modify our behaviour so as to limit the dose to ourselves and our families.

As far as the authorities are concerned, one of their first priorities should be to prevent radiation doses to the public or indeed to any occupationally exposed workers being anywhere near those that cause immediately detectable physical effects. As we have seen earlier, these effects are those which appear only after a fairly high radiation dose has been delivered, and they are caused by acute doses delivered in a short period of time, as distinct to prolonged ones.

By comparison long-term chronic effects, for instance cancers, tend not to be seen or felt for years. The danger is that authorities will underplay the risks associated with radiation as a cause of cancers and other life-shortening effects simply because tangible proof of the association is open to widely different interpretations.

·✦✦✦·· The accident at Three Mile Island ··✦✦✦·

The worst accident so far in a pressurized water reactor (PWR) happened in the United States at Three Mile Island on 28 March 1979, with the reactor operating at very nearly full power. It occurred when a pump to the steam generators stopped working and the back-up pump also failed. Through a series of blunders, including an essential signal lamp being hidden by a maintenance tag, and because various valves stuck open, the coolant water was lost from the reactor core. Hot uranium fuel was exposed, over-heated and crumbled, releasing explosive hydrogen gas and highly radioactive fission products. Luckily, the ensuing hydrogen explosion did not burst the concrete containment. It was fortunate too that the only radioactive substances to escape into the environment were some 17 curies of radio-iodine and up to 13 million curies of inert gases such as argon and krypton.

The initial concern of the scientists and technicians juggling with the reactor was to prevent molten pieces of the core bursting the reactor pressure-vessel and destroying the containment. However the accident did not finish there. By November 1979, six months later, the base of the containment building was flooded to a depth of six feet and highly radioactive water was still leaking in at the rate of 1,000 gallons a day, threatening vital electrical equipment.

In June 1980, the United States Nuclear Regulatory Commission decided that krypton gas still trapped in the building should be vented into the atmosphere. The decision led to vehement protests from the population in the surrounding area, but the NRC justified it on the grounds that even greater risks would arise unless their staff were able to gain access.

A month later they began to release the krypton through a tall chimney – some 2,000 people opted to leave the area while the operation was in progress – and on 23 July two engineers clad in protective clothing and using special respirators briefly entered the containment building.

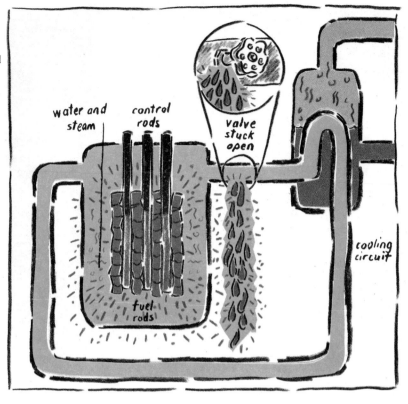

Three Mile Island: water and steam leaking out of a stuck open valve caused the reactor to overheat and the fuel to melt down. A massive hydrogen explosion was narrowly averted.

water and steam

control rods

valve stuck open

cooling circuit

fuel rods

The big clean-up

In the following months, the experts charged with the task of cleaning up the site gradually began to realize the full magnitude of the challenge that faced them. In August 1979, the operators believed that they would have the reactor 'back in business' by the middle of 1983. The cost of the entire job was estimated to be $400 million.

In December 1980, however, they announced that the clean-up could not be completed before mid-1985 and that it would cost at least $1,000 million. The task of removing the highly radioactive debris proved exceedingly difficult and was still only one-fifth completed by the end of 1986, and new problems are still emerging.

Counting the cost

The cost, too, has been formidable. With 2,500 workers on site, all of whom must be continually rotated to new jobs as their radiation dosage reaches the permitted maximum, the payroll alone was recently running at between $30 and $40 million a year. This figure looks set to rise rather than to fall, because the estimated number of man-hours required to complete the job has since been revised upwards by a factor of six.

The Japanese nuclear industry, conscious, no doubt, that its own fortunes were inextricably tied up with the safety of PWRs, also contributed $18 million and the services of 20 scientists and engineers. By the end of 1986, some $700 million had already been spent.

Accidents – how often and how bad?

In 1975 the United States Nuclear Regulatory Commission carried out a study on the probabilities and consequences of accidents occurring in light water reactors then operating. The Commission concluded that the chance of a major accident was likely to be 1 in every 1,000 million years of reactor operation: a highly improbable event. The team of scientists nevertheless agreed that a major escape of radioactive materials from a full-sized reactor might lead to 45,000 deaths, 250,000 injuries, and damage to property worth $124,000 million upwards.

To measure probabilities, the scientists had used the technique known as fault tree analysis, in which the consequences of each malfunction and its likelihood are followed through to a logical conclusion. A major criticism of such methodology is that it fails completely to take account of a 'multiple mode failure', in which several separately functioning parts break down simultaneously. In 1975, for instance, a fire in a cable channel started by workmen searching for air leaks with a candle destroyed the control systems of two twin reactors at the Browns Ferry plant in Alabama. Luckily both reactors responded to manual control and were shut down, yet the incident could have led to a common mode failure. The Three Mile Island accident also involved common mode failure, and it came uncomfortably close to the 1 in 1,000 million probability.

⚜ Accident at Chernobyl ⚜

At 1.23 am on the morning of Saturday 26 April 1986, a powerful explosion inside the Number 4 reactor at the Chernobyl nuclear power station in the Ukraine blew aside the 1,000-tonne lid of a massive steel vessel and blasted through the surrounding concrete containment structure. Bits of graphite, chunks of uranium fuel and pieces of control rods were strewn around the reactor building. The red-hot graphite still inside the reactor burst into flames as air rushed in, and like coke in a blast furnace it began to burn vigorously.

Two men died in the first moments of the blast, one from falling masonry and one from burns. Over the following months some 30 others were to die, most of them firemen who battled heroically to prevent the fire from spreading to the reactor in the next building. All died from radiation burns and radiation sickness following exposure to strong gamma and beta radiation from the broken reactor core. In addition to radiation from outside their bodies, some had also been exposed to large internal doses from breathing in radioactive particles.

Over the next few days the Soviet authorities marshalled their resources to evacuate 135,000 people, all of whom lived within 30 kilometres (19 miles) of the power station – an area of nearly 3,000 square kilometres (1,100 square miles). Livestock had to be moved, and attempts were made to control the contamination that was settling out by covering soil and buildings alike.

Meanwhile the fire in the reactor had to be put out, and the reactor itself smothered to prevent the escape of even more radioactive material. Helicopters, flying 24 hours a day, were used to dump 5,000 tonnes of material onto the burning core. This included some 800 tonnes of dolomite – a limestone rock – to generate carbon dioxide gas to quench the fire; boron carbide – a neutron absorber – to ensure that the nuclear chain reaction remained shut down; 2,400 tonnes of lead to blanket the exposed core and absorb gamma radiation; and 1,800 tonnes of clay and sand to help to seal off the fire. The strategy worked and by 6 May the temperature of the core had fallen, and the release of radioactive materials dropped sharply. The Soviets believed that beween 30 million and 50 million curies of radioactive substances escaped, amounting in all to a few per cent of the total inventory of the core. Moreover, it was the more voltaile substances such as iodine and caesium that escaped in relatively large quantites, while inert gases such as krypton and xenon escaped in their entirety. The estimate is that 20 per cent of the radio-iodine was lost from core, and approximately 12 per cent of the radio-caesium. It was these substances in particular that later fell-out over much of Europe, contaminating food and water supplies.

Nevertheless, fall-out was sufficiently high over the first couple of weeks after the explosion that many thousands of people received substantial radiation doses through gamma and beta radiation. The Soviets used a comparatively large dose as a criterion for evacuation. They now state that the official annual limit for individual exposure to radiation is 5 rems (50 millisieverts), which is ten times the ICRP limit and equivalent to more than 25 times the natural background radiation dose. Even so, towards the end of May some villages and small towns in Byelorussia several hundred kilometres away from Chernobyl had to be evacuated, in addition to those in the 30-kilometre zone around the stricken reactor.

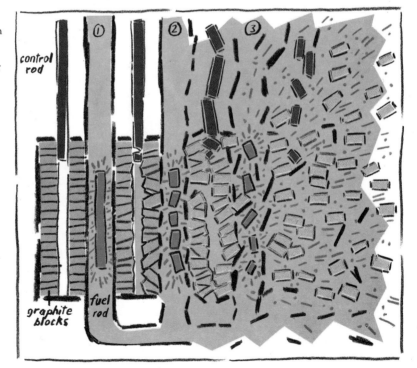

Chernobyl: the accident occurred when steam built up around the fuel, making the chain reaction go faster and faster. The increase in heat generated more steam until the fuel fragmented, causing a massive steam and hydrogen explosion. Graphite bricks and fuel fragments were hurled through the destroyed reactor containment.

What went wrong at Chernobyl?

The Chernobyl disaster was a profound shock to the nuclear industry. Although it was conceptually possible that a reactor could blow up in this way, nuclear engineers believed that they had incorporated enough safety precautions and back-up systems into their designs that a nuclear runaway accident was virtually impossible. Indeed the proability of an accident of this type was put in the order of one for every 10 million or even every 100 million years of reactor operation – an almost negligible risk. And whereas the public may have got used to hearing about core meltdowns, because of the partial meltdown at Three Mile Island in Pennsylvania, it had been assured that a nuclear power station could not explode – and certainly not like an atomic bomb. Yet the explosion at Chernobyl was the result of a runaway chain reaction of the kind that – in a millionth of that time – creates an atomic bomb explosion. In addition the fall-out from Chernobyl was many times greater, possibly by a factor of a thousand, than would occur after a Hiroshima-sized atomic bomb blast.

In fact, the reactor core at Chernobyl disrupted after a surge in the chain reaction took the power to several hundred times the normal operating level. In a remarkably candid account to a meeting of the International Atomic Energy Agency held at its headquarters in Vienna in August 1986, the Soviet delegation stated that the prime cause of the accident was a number of violations of operational practice by technicians at the plant. Ironically, they had set out to test a system for improving plant safety.

Reactors tend to be unstable when operated at low power, one reason being that the amount of the neutron-absorber xenon-135 becomes significantly large in proportion to the numbers of neutrons that are available for sustaining the chain reaction. Unfortunately in the experiment that led to the disaster, the technicians let the power fall too far (down to some 7 per cent of full power), at which point they had to juggle with the reactor controls to prevent the reactor shutting down altogether.

As the operators continued manipulating the controls, the chain reaction slowly began to build up, so raising the power and generating more heat. The water began to flash into steam – a process that in itself tended to make more neutrons available for the chain reaction. Within seconds, the operators were confronted with a runaway situation, with the power building up to more than a thousand times of what it had been moments before. They tried to scram the reactor by dropping in the control rods, but by then they had been raised a long way out of the core and needed many seconds to become fully inserted – far too slow to stop the reaction that had already been unleashed. The resulting explosion blew the fuel apart, and effectively brought the chain reaction to a violent end.

Radiation escape from Chernobyl continued throughout the first week and into the second. Heavy rain over parts of Scandinavia and western Europe washed out considerable quantities of radioactive substances. Some of these areas received several hundred times the fall-out compared with regions remaining dry. Radio-iodine and radio-caesium were by far the most significant isotopes. Milk products and vegetables were quickly contaminated. In places such as Gävle, 100 kilometres (about 60 miles) north of Stockholm and several thousand kilometres away from Chernobyl, the fall-out levels were so high that livestock had to be kept indoors for several months. Hay and silage made from contaminated pasture concentrated the fall-out, later leading to problems with winter feeding of livestock. Indeed in many parts of Europe where fall-out had been high, as in Bavaria in West Germany, levels of radioactive contamination rose again in winter because cattle were being fed with contaminated hay and silage.

In Britain, heavy rain over North Wales, Cumbria and Scotland led to a surprisingly high deposition of radio-caesium. Sheep in particular became contaminated, and many thousand lambs about to be slaughtered for meat were found to have caesium levels in excess of 1,000 becquerels per kilogram, the level set by the British government as the upper limit for sale and consumption. The British Ministry of Agriculture, Food and Fisheries had expected the levels to fall over the lamb-growing season but had miscalculated; the ban was lifted (and then only partly) at the end of February 1987, 10 months after the initial fall-out. In fact some 500,000 sheep remained on the 'restricted list' throughout 1987.

Undoubtedly the people worse affected outside the Soviet Union were the Lapps – the Sami people – of the northern parts of Norway, Sweden and Finland, who live almost exclusively off reindeer and their products. There again radiation levels showed a marked rise towards the end of winter. According to a Swedish National Radio report of 2 February 1987, the radioactivity level in reindeer had risen to 42,000 becquerels per kilogram – more than six times its September average of around 6,600 becquerels per kilogram. The situation for the Sami is particularly acute because the lichens on which reindeer feed retain their contamination for several years. The reproductivity of the animals is also bound to be affected by such high levels of radiation.

When to warn the public

After a nuclear accident, the authorities have to decide what action to take and what to recommend to the public. What needs to be known is how a certain level of a radionuclide such as caesium-137 – in the air, on the ground or in the water supply – is likely to behave in terms of its getting into the food chain and ultimately into human beings. For instance, if there is a particular amount of caesium deposited on the ground, what does that mean in terms of dose to us? How much radiation will we get simply from external gamma radiation? And if the caesium is on pasture, how much will get into the meat of animals and how much into milk and other dairy products?

With those fundamental questions in mind, and appreciating that an accident situation demands a relatively swift analysis, authorities such as Britain's NRPB have drawn up what are termed Derived Emergency Reference Levels (DERLs). For instance, a particular amount of a radio-isotope on pasture translates into such-and-such a dose to infants, 10-year old children or adults. Two levels of action are recommended, a lower and upper, for each category of countermeasure. Thus, at a dose equivalent of 50 millisieverts to the thyroid gland, the authorities should be seriously considering whether the public ought to be given stable iodine tablets to prevent the uptake into the thyroid of radio-iodine. By the time the dose has been put at 250 millisieverts action should already have been taken.

An estimated dose of 5 millisieverts to the whole body, or 50 millisieverts to the skin, thyroid, lungs or other individual organs, ought to have alerted the authorities to the eventuality that the public should take shelter. Once those doses have reached 25 millisieverts to the whole body and 250 millisieverts to any one organ, shelter should already have been prescribed.

Evacuation, on the other hand, should be seriously considered when the radiation dose to the whole body is estimated to be reaching 100 millisieverts, or equally the dose to the thyroid or to any other individual organ has reached 300 millisieverts and to the skin 1,000 millisieverts. By the time the dose to the whole body would have got to 500 millisieverts, or 1,500 to an individual organ or 5,000 millisieverts to the skin, we should already have been evacuated.

The Derived Emergency Reference Level is therefore a way of carrying out relatively simple measurements of radiation in the air and on the ground and of coming to conclusions as to the severity of the radiation exposure should no action be taken. The problem is to get the balance right: excessively hasty action would cause enormous disruption, while waiting to be told what to do may put us all at unneccessary risk. In effect, we have to decide whether or not we can fully trust those authorities in charge of dealing with nuclear accidents. Are they doing the measurements properly and are they letting us know the results?

Undoubtedly one of the worst aspects of a nuclear accident is its psychological effect. We cannot see the plume and we cannot immediately feel it in terms of its effect on our bodies. In the end we may want to know for ourselves how high the radiation levels are around us.

In fact, a simple geiger counter, preferably one which totals up the number of counts over a set period of time, gives a fair idea of the amount of gamma radiation around us – for instance, in the air and on the ground. It does not tell us what radioactive elements are causing the high radiation levels nor will it indicate whether alpha emitters such as plutonium have also been released. Nonetheless, armed with a geiger counter and with some experience in using it, we should be able to judge for ourselves something of the severity of the accident in terms of radiation releases. The great advantage of having a geiger counter is that it may help to put our minds at rest should we decide to stay put. Equally it should alert us to the possibility that the authorities are prevaricating and are not keeping us properly informed.

An ordinary geiger counter is a relatively crude piece of equipment in terms of what it can do. Should we want to know more specifically what is in the plume and what is falling out around us, then we need the results of a more exhaustive analysis, which is best carried out by specialists in a laboratory.

Governments have their own monitoring stations for radioactivity. Nuclear power plants are also equipped with sophisticated measuring and monitoring systems as are many universities and technical colleges. What undoubtedly has been lacking to date is a well-coordinated system that operates wholeheartedly in the public interest. However, following the disaster at Chernobyl, in the UK for example, the NRPB (The National Radiological Protection Board) has suggested using the monitoring resources available in a nationwide network co-ordinated by itself. It remains to be seen whether it will be successful.

Variable fall-out

One of the main surprises of Chernobyl was the way that fall-out levels could vary by a factor of ten or more over a short distance. The highest levels were where it had rained heavily, yet the fact of it raining was not enough in itself to cause high radiation levels on the ground. This happened only when the actual mass of contaminated air was passing underneath the rain cloud. Indeed, it was later determined that most radioactivity had been washed out of the plume by rain falling from above it.

The differences were indeed remarkable. In France, for example, both the Atomic Energy Commission and Electricité de France (EdF) took measurements of Chernobyl fall-out near their nuclear installations. Cadarache, for instance, is a nuclear installation belonging to the CEA, France's Atomic Energy Commission. During the period when the Chernobyl plume was over France between 1 and 5 May 1986, the maximum radiation concentration in the air close to Cadarache was found to be 18.5 becquerels per cubic metre. Meanwhile Cadarache received just 10 millimetres (less than half an inch) of rain at that time and the fall-out levels on the ground were measured at 14,200 becquerels per square metre.

Cruas is an EdF nuclear power site some 100 kilometres (63 miles) away from Cadarache. There the maximum air concentration was 8.7 becquerels per cubic metre. However, it rained heavily – more than 30 millimetres (1.2 inches) over those few crucial days – and the deposition on the ground was 250,000 becquerels per square metre. This was almost 20 times more than at Cadarache, despite the air concentration being less than half, demonstrating the importance of weather conditions.

Obviously, unless every locality is measured for fall-out, some areas will be entirely missed (especially in the countryside) and the people who live there left in ignorance. What Chernobyl taught us was that we should be on our guard if it rains heavily at a time when the radioactive cloud is somewhere in the vicinity. We therefore need to know the meteorological conditions and have some idea of the whereabouts of the main mass of radioactively contaminated air. And until we are advised to the contrary,

The plume's progress: following a nuclear accident the heaviest fall-out is likely to occur closest to the reactor. However, places much further away may get heavily doused with fall-out when rain washes through the radioactive plume.

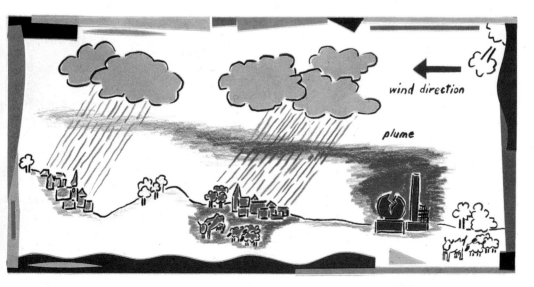

wind direction

plume

we should not drink fresh rainwater, stay out in the rain or, once the rain has stopped, go for a swim in an open swimming pool.

Perhaps, in all of western Europe, France's official attitude to the Chernobyl fall-out was the most reprehensible: perhaps not so suprising given the very large commitment to nuclear power. For instance, on 6 May 1986, just after France had received extensive fall-out from Chernobyl in parts of the east and west of the country, the Ministry of Agriculture stated categorically that France 'by dint of its distance (from the Ukraine) had been completely spared from the fall-out of Chernobyl'. A few days later, Professor Pierre Pellerin, the director of France's SCPRI (Service Central de Protection contre les Rayonnements Ionisants) admitted some contamination had taken place: nevertheless the levels given were far below those actually received. According to the SCPRI, the 252,000 becquerels per square metre on the ground near Cruas translated into 37,000 – therefore seven times less.

Corsica – a case of deceit

The role of the SCPRI in France is equivalent to that of the NRPB in Britain, in so far as it is to protect the public against the effects of excessive discharges of radioactive substances, whether they be routine releases from nuclear installations or a result of accidents. The SCPRI should therefore inform and advise as to what measures ought to be taken for the general public so as to mitigate the effects of ionizing radiation. In France, following the Chernobyl accident, the SCPRI was so keen to keep the public in ignorance that as a result people were exposed unnecessarily to radiation. Had proper advice been given much of the worst exposure could have been avoided.

SCPRI's negligence was particularly evident in Corsica. In a bulletin of 2 June 1986, Professor Pellerin published two charts indicating the meteorology and weather conditions affecting France and Corsica between 29 April and 5 May. Indeed, at the end of April and beginning of May the radioactive cloud was seen to be over Corsica, having passed over Italy. While the Italian authorities imposed restrictions on the consumption of fresh milk

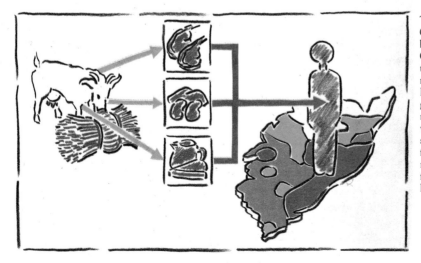

The eastern part of Corsica was badly hit by the fall-out from Chernobyl. Initially the problem was from radio-iodine, but a long-term problem was generated by radioactive caesium which was picked up by sheep and goats both from foraging in the mountain pastures and from contaminated hay.

and vegetables in the northern part of the country, the French authorities turned a blind eye and left the Corsicans in ignorance.

The first actual official measurements of contamination in Corsica were carried out on 12 May 1986. The Corsicans, particularly in the mountain areas, use sheep's milk both for drinking and to make soft cheeses which are eaten within a couple of days of manufacture. Sheep's milk on 12 May gave a reading of 4,400 becquerels per litre of iodine-131, 160 becquerels per litre of caesium-134, and 410 becquerels of caesium-137. (These readings are equivalent to 2,500, 91 and 233 bequerels per pint, respectively.)

Iodine-131 has a physical half-life of just over 8 days, and each day the activity present on the ground and on the pasture falls by a factor of 0.917. Because the fall-out from the Chernobyl cloud over Corsica took place at the beginning of May, going back in time from 12 May meant that originally sheep's milk would have had close to 15,000 becquerels per litre (more than 8,500 becquerels per pint).

In fact, the European Commission made recommendations to member countries of the Common Market that milk with an iodine-131 content higher than 500 becquerels per litre, on 6 May, should be banned from immediate consumption, with a maximum of 250 becquerels per litre on 16 May and 125 becquerels per litre on 26 May. The reason for a falling permissible level is based on the assumption that milk is consumed as normal during the period of contamination, and that if all the successive doses from iodine-131 are added up they will give a total quantity that does not exceed the recommended annual dose limits.

As it happened, none of the member Common Market countries accepted the European Commission's recommendations precisely as given, but even France with an upper limit of 3,700 becquerels per litre was far below what must have been the level of iodine-131 contamination in Corsican sheep's milk. All the other European countries went for tougher restrictions. Britain decided to stick with the 2,000 becquerels per litre indicated in its Derived Emergency Reference Levels. Nevertheless, as the NRPB pointed out, the DERLs were prescribed on the basis that the releases of radionuclides in a reactor accident took place in one burst rather than over a succession of days, and that the 2,000 becquerels per litre was a peak dose followed by dwindling doses after that as a result of both the physical decay of iodine-131 and its elimination from the milking animal. The DERL for milk was obtained on the basis that a year's consumption of some 260 litres by a one-year old child would give a dose to the thyroid of 50 millisieverts, equivalent to a whole-body dose of 1.7 millisieverts.

The other European countries considered the British level to be too lax. West Germany and the Netherlands decided that bans on consumption should be imposed for levels above 500 becquerels per litre, and many of the West German States went even further, with Hessen for example deciding that anything above 20 becquerels per litre would be too high. Italy actually put the bans in force for children under the age of 10 and for pregnant women to last for the first couple of weeks in May 1986.

Estimates indicate that an initial fall-out on the ground of 13,000 becquerels per square metre on pasture land will transfer into 2,000 becquerels per litre of iodine-131 in cow's milk. However those calculations are based on British pasture conditions with cows as the grazing animals. Conditions in the mountains of Corsica involving both aromatic plants and poorer grasses with sheep as the grazing animals are substantially different.

Whereas a cow passes approximately 1 per cent of the iodine-131 taken into its body each day into every litre of milk, therefore some ten per cent total in 10 litres of milk each day (approx 2 gallons per day); a ewe passes on a total of approximately 30 per cent and a goat 5 per cent in a much smaller volume of milk. Furthermore, aromatic plants such as those found in the Mediterranean mountains, growing on poor soils, tend to concentrate into themselves minerals that have fallen with rain. The combination of these two factors puts consumers of sheep's milk at particular risk should there be radioactive fall-out.

What sort of doses would the community in Corsica have received on the basis that nobody took precautions? The traditional diet in the hills consists of fresh vegetables and dairy products. A child of five, for instance, consumes at least 200 grams (7 ounces) of fresh sheep's cheese each day as well as drinking milk. At least 5 litres (nearly 8 pints) of fresh milk go into the making of 1 kilogram (2.2 pounds) of fresh cheese, and most of the radioactivity, whether iodine or caesium, stays with the curds rather than passing into the whey. The minimum daily consumption of milk, whether fresh or in the form of a day-old cheese, would be 1 litre (1.76 pints) for such a child and likely more for an older child or an adult.

Through knowing how much ingested iodine-131 gets into the thyroid gland compared with the amount excreted from the body, scientists have made estimates of the likely dose to the thyroid for each becquerel. The thyroid of a young person, although smaller than that of an adult, is very active and for a given intake into the body receives a higher dose. The NRPB, for instance, estimates that a becquerel of iodine-131 will give a dose to the thyroid of 3.7 millionths of a sievert, one-third of that to a 10-year old child, and approximately one-ninth to an adult. Other authorities use similar numbers, the West Germans adding a number for 5 year-olds

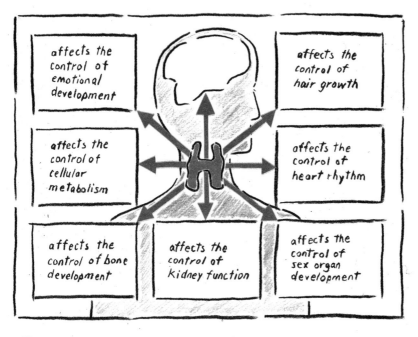

affects the control of emotional development

affects the control of hair growth

affects the control of cellular metabolism

affects the control of heart rhythm

affects the control of bone development

affects the control of kidney function

affects the control of sex organ development

The thyroid gland has many functions especially in growing children. Following a reactor accident the danger is that the thyroid will accumulate damaging levels of radioactive iodine.

of approximately 2 millionths of a sievert per becquerel. Thus 15,000 becquerels per litre peak dose followed by a fall-off in dose as the radio-iodine decays away, as received by some Corsican children, will give a thyroid dose over the course of the year of 375 millisieverts and a whole-body dose of nearly 13 millisieverts – more than five times the natural background dose. Young children are at risk not only because of their ability to concentrate iodine in the thyroid but also because healthy growth depends crucially on the proper function of the gland. The thyroid thus regulates the growth of bones and cartilage in the joints, helps control cellular metabolism, including the regulation of body temperature, influences cardiac rhythm, is crucial for the development of the gonads in both sexes and has important psychic and emotional effects. Young children must therefore comprise the critical group in any evaluation of risk from radioactive fall-out.

The foetus is particularly sensitive to the effects of radio-iodine. Studies indicate that a three-month-old foetus will concentrate iodine a hundred times more than an adult and more than three times more than a one-year-old baby.

✦✦✦ Contamination of livestock ✦✦✦

Because they are out in the open, livestock are particularly at risk. In one heavily contaminated area in Corsica, approximately a third of all cows in calf at the time of Chernobyl lost their calves. In Bavaria, the calf mortality rate among exposed cattle increased as much as four-fold.

The Federal Authorities in West Germany had recommended that cattle be kept under cover at least until 11 May. In Bavaria one group of organic farmers decided to continue keeping their cattle under cover, even though the restrictions had been lifted. The animals were therefore entirely free of contaminated forage, at least during those critical first weeks. An investigation into the mortality of calves born over the next autumn and winter revealed that five had been still-born out of 214 births, a percentage of 2.3 per cent and in marked contrast to the 7.1 average percentage for stillbirths in Bavaria.

Meanwhile, for cattle as a whole in Bavaria the number of artifical inseminations performed to achieve preganancy tripled in the months following the Chernobyl fall-out, an indication that the spontaneous abortion rate had risen.

Direct contamination of humans
Radioactivity in the air can harm us directly through irradiation of the skin and body, either through gamma radiation from a metre or more away or from radionuclides that deposit on our hair, face, hands and clothes. We are also likely to breathe in radioactive substances, some of which may become lodged in the lungs, or get absorbed into the bloodstream.

As far as the authorities are concerned, a close watch has to be kept over the air concentrations of radio-isotopes in the immediate aftermath of an accident to see whether they are high enough to warrant evacuation of people, or at least sheltering. The authorities must therefore estimate

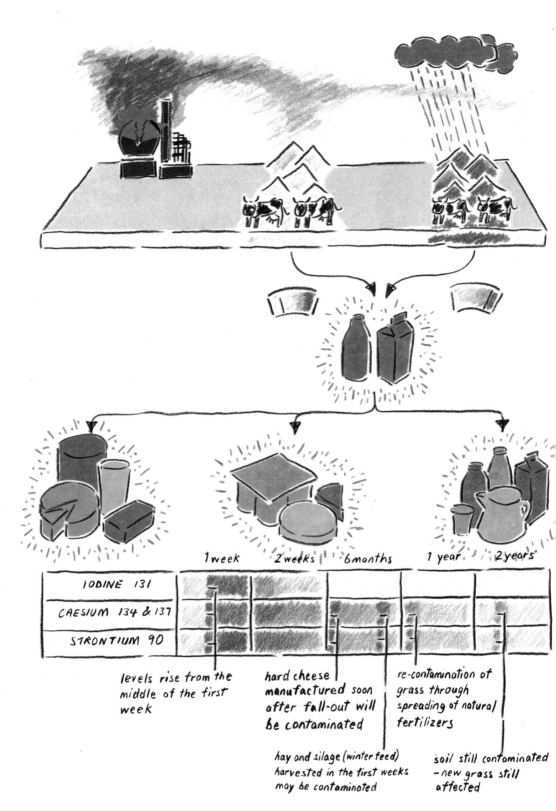

	1 week	2 weeks	6 months	1 year	2 years
IODINE 131					
CAESIUM 134 & 137					
STRONTIUM 90					

levels rise from the middle of the first week

hard cheese manufactured soon after fall-out will be contaminated

re-contamination of grass through spreading of natural fertilizers

hay and silage (winter feed) harvested in the first weeks may be contaminated

soil still contaminated – new grass still affected

The fall-out deposited during dry conditions is ten or even 100 times less compared with that when it rains heavily through the plume. Higher fall-out will be reflected in heavier contamination of milk and dairy products. In good fertile soils the caesium is quickly bound and kept out of harms way. In poor soils the caesium remains mobile and available to plants.

whether integrated doses to the skin, lungs and whole body from both internal and external radiation sources are likely over the days following the accident to lead to effective individual doses of 100 millisieverts or more. The NRPB gives a DERL for iodine-131 in the air of 2,300 million becquerels per cubic metre per second as being indicative that evacuation should be seriously considered. The critical person is taken as a child of 10 years-old. Obviously not just one radio-isotope will be present in the air, and the activities of all the major radioactive components must be taken into account. That such high activities can arise is evident from the need of the Soviet authorities to evacuate the immediate area around Chernobyl within the first 48 hours following the explosion. Despite that evacuation, a number of people in the nearby town of Pripyat received estimated whole-body doses of 500 millisieverts or more.

Even with evacuation, all people exposed to relatively high concentrations of radioactive iodine should take tablets of stable iodine at a prescribed rate to swamp the thyroid gland and prevent uptake of the radioactive isotope. On the other hand, iodine tablets should not be taken unless absolutely necessary because some people can suffer a toxic reaction and become extremely sick.

Those who are farther away from the radioactive plume and have been informed that it is likely to come their way may consider less draconian measures than taking iodide tablets to build up their stable iodine levels in the body. One way is to consume a sprinkling of Japanese seaweed (kelp) over one's food, or take kelp tablets (the seaweed contains natural iodine). For protection an adult needs to take some 20 milligrams of iodide every three days while the danger of high radio-iodine levels remain. A young child should take ten times less.

CHAPTER
⚜ 5 ⚜

Food and environment

For collecting and concentrating radioactive fall-out deposited on pasture it would be difficult to devise a more effective mechanism than a herd of grazing animals. Cattle, sheep, goats and deer forage over wide areas and ingest the fall-out that coats the surfaces of plants in the days immediately following the passage of the plume – both by swallowing it and by breathing it in. Furthermore, they subsequently continue to accumulate radioactive substances after these have found their way into the food plants (which absorb them directly or take them up from the soil along with other minerals). With four radio-isotopes in particular, a significant proportion of the fall-out is passed on in the animals' milk.

The four isotopes whose presence in milk can pose a serious threat to consumers are iodine-131, caesium-137, caesium-134 and strontium-90. Iodine, being the most volatile, is the one most likely to be released in the largest quantities in the event of an accident. It is estimated, for example, that about 20 per cent of the iodine in the core of the Chernobyl reactor (some 700,000 million million becquerels) escaped into the environment, while the corresponding figures for caesium and strontium were 10 per cent (50,000 million million becquerels) and 4 per cent (about 20,000 million million becquerels). It does not necessarily follow, however, that if the plume contains given proportions of the three substances, they will be deposited in the same proportions. The Chernobyl accident showed us, for instance, that while ten times more iodine is deposited when the fall-out is 'washed out' of the plume by rain rather than falling as 'dry deposition', rain causes the deposition of caesium to increase a hundredfold.

Obviously, because all three elements are likely to be present in contaminated milk, it is essential to take account of their cumulative effects when assessing the risks. But their characteristics are very different, and should be considered separately.

The most important point about iodine-131 is that it has a relatively short half-life of only 8 days. This means that although it poses very serious dangers in the immediate aftermath of an accident, those dangers diminish fairly rapidly and some steps can be made to avert them – or at least minimize the risks. It may, for example, be possible for farmers to keep their animals indoors and feed them on stored fodder that contains little or no contamination. It also means that even if fresh milk contains very high levels of radio-iodine, products made from that milk, such as hard cheese (which takes time to mature) or butter (which can be stored for long periods of time), may nonetheless become perfectly safe to eat.

On the other hand, many dairy products are normally eaten within a matter of days or even hours, and these may be particularly dangerous because the manufacturing processes actually concentrate the iodine present in milk. Soft cheeses, for instance, are often eaten within two days of manufacture, and although one-fifth of the radio-iodine will have decayed over that period, this is more than offset by the fact that it takes 4-5 litres (7-9 pints) of milk to make 1 kilogram (2.2 pounds) of cheese, and that virtually all the iodine is concentrated in the curds rather than being discarded along with the whey.

So far as our bodies are concerned, iodine-131 is indistinguishable from ordinary iodine, an element that is essential to our health and which is normally concentrated in the thyroid gland. The risks associated with iodine-131 are therefore calculated in terms of the radiation dose that is likely to be delivered to the thyroid as a result of swallowing contaminated food and/or breathing contaminated air. These risks are considerably higher for children, partly because they absorb up to ten times more iodine than an adult given a similar level of intake, and partly because the thyroid plays a crucial role in regulating growth. Damage to the organ can result in serious developmental problems.

Opinions about what constitutes a 'safe' level of iodine in milk (and elsewhere) have had to be revised in the wake of the Chernobyl disaster. Most calculations had previously been based on the assumption that any release of radioactive materials into the atmosphere would take place within a matter of hours at most. It was therefore assumed that even if some people received a high initial dose of iodine, the substance's rapid rate of decay would ensure that nobody was subjected to a high dose rate for a prolonged period.

But at Chernobyl fission products continued to pour out into the atmosphere for ten days (and, at much reduced rates, for even longer), with only 25 per cent of the total release occurring on the first day. As a result, iodine levels remained high for far longer than anybody had foreseen. In Stockholm, for example, the level of radio-iodine in the air reached 11

Cattle, sheep and goats, by grazing over large areas of ground, will concentrate radioactive fall-out in their bodies and in their milk. How much radioactivity gets into milk products such as cheese, butter, yogurt and cream depends on the type of radioactivity and the processing required in making the milk product.

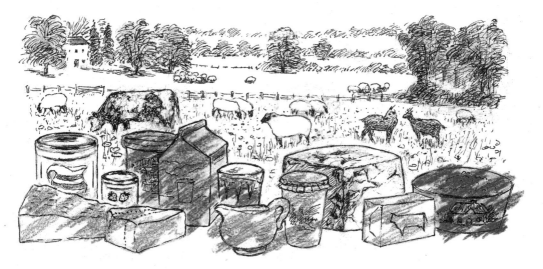

becquerels per cubic metre three days after the accident. Two days later, the original plume having passed on, the level had fallen to just one-tenth of a becquerel per cubic metre, but it then rose steadily over the following week to reach a new peak of 2 becquerels per cubic metre before finally falling away again.

Stockholm was by no means the worst affected place. In eastern Bavaria and parts of south-western Germany along the frontier with France, four days after the accident each cubic metre of air contained, on average, 170 becquerels of radio-iodine. An adult, breathing in about 20 cubic metres of air a day, could therefore absorb up to 3,400 becquerels from this source alone.

A cow has a lung capacity about eight times larger than that of a human being, and can therefore absorb as much as 24,000 becquerels of iodine each day simply by breathing in air that contains 150 becquerels per cubic metre. Under these conditions, each litre of milk taken from the animal could be expected to contain 240 becquerels – enough to give a dose of 120 microsieverts to the thyroid of an adult. The same litre of milk could deliver a dose of 960 microsieverts – almost 1 millisievert – to the thyroid of a child. Just that one litre of milk therefore could give the child an effective whole-body dose equal to a tenth of that now recommended as the maximum dose for a whole year. In similar circumstances, a sheep or goat, both of which have an air intake much smaller than that of a cow (but also gives far less milk), might be expected to produce milk containing about 135 becquerels per litre.

In many circumstances – especially when the radioactive substances are washed out of the plume by rain – the amounts of fall-out that animals breathe in are far less significant than those they pick up with their food. In the same area of south-western Germany, for example, a violent thunderstorm occurred in early May, a few days after the accident at Chernobyl, and samples of grass subsequently taken from pastureland were found to contain 6,000 becquerels of radio-iodine per kilogram. A cow consuming a daily ration of 55 kilograms (about 100 pounds) of fodder containing a somewhat lower level of contamination – say 4,000 becquerels per kilogram – might still produce milk with more than 2,000 becquerels per litre. In fact, the highest level of radio-iodine contamination found in milk in West Germany was 1,500 becquerels per litre. In Britain, levels never rose above 50 becquerels per litre in the south, where the weather remained dry, and 400 becquerels in the north, where there was a good deal of rain.

To put these figures in persepective, they should be compared with the recommended maximums adopted by various countries in the aftermath of Chernobyl. In Britain the National Radiological Protection Board (NRPB) recommended that milk could continue to be sold as long as it contained no more than 2,000 becquerels of radio-iodine per litre. This calculation is based on the premise that iodine levels would decline rapidly, and that the maximum acceptable dose to the thyroid over the course of one year should be set at 50 millisieverts. The French were apparently more sanguine, setting the maximum acceptable level of contamination at 3,700 becquerels per litre – although this figure included all radioactive substances, not just radio-iodine. But West Germany, the Netherlands and Belgium were far more cautious and banned the sale of milk containing more than 500 becquerels of iodine per litre. At that level, an adult would have to drink two-thirds of a litre of milk every day for a year before reaching the 50 millisievert thyroid dose. It is difficult to think of any circumstances in which such high levels of iodine contamination would continue for so long. On the other hand, a ten-year-old child consuming a litre of milk a day (1.75 pints) at the level adopted by the British could receive the 'safe' maximum dose in just over one month.

As well as maximum permissible levels for the contamination of milk itself, a ban is also imposed on all consumption of milk from areas where the actual fall-out of iodine reaches a certain amount. In Britain, for example, the NRPB has recommended that children should not drink milk if the deposition of radio-iodine on pastureland exceeds 13,000 becquerels per square metre, and that the ban should be extended to adults if the deposition exceeds 98,000 becquerels per square metre.

Caesium and strontium in milk
Once they have been ingested by grazing animals, caesium and strontium also pass into their milk. Estimates indicate that up to 15 per cent of the caesium and 6 per cent of the radioactive strontium ingested finish up in the milk. For caesium, levels of up to 10,000 becquerels per kilogram were measured in hay cut in the Drome region of France in mid-June 1986, one-and-a-half months after the Chernobyl accident. On average, a milking ewe or goat gives 2 litres of milk a day. So if it eats 2 kilograms of contaminated hay a day, 1,500 becquerels per litre will turn up in its milk. A one-year-old child consuming up to 0.7 litres a day of such milk (as milk or soft cheese) for 4 months would receive a whole-body dose of 9.4 millisieverts – far above the acceptable limit of 0.5 millisieverts.

Meat

Animals, like human beings, can become irradiated with fall-out by breathing in radioactive aerosols or particles, by ingesting contaminated food, and through direct external radiation from substances on the ground and on their skin. Animals exposed to very high levels of radiation suffer from radiation sickness and without the kind of treatment that can be afforded to humans usually die.

Our main concern, however, is not with the health of animals but with the level of radioactive contamination in meat and other animal products. Unless the animals are close to the source of radiation, they are more likely to be affected by fall-out on the ground and on vegetation than by radioactive material carried in the plume. Therefore, although in the short term animals may breathe in relatively large quantities of radioisotopes such as iodine from the plume, the more important long-term contamination is from ingesting food, especially in areas where it has rained heavily.

Sheltering the animals while the plume is passing and keeping them in for several weeks (if possible) effectively reduces exposure to some of the shorter-lived radio-isotopes such as iodine-131. Yet the length of time that shelter and supplementary feeding can be continued is obviously limited, especially during the summer months.

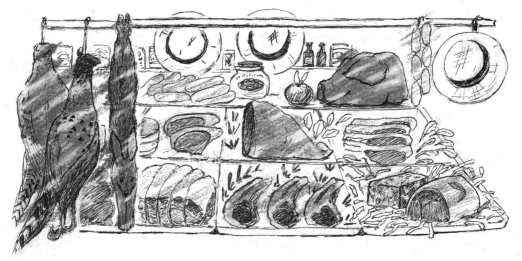

Contamination of winter feed – particularly hay and silage – can also be a problem. Even if the animals are kept off grazing land, the same crop made into winter feed will contain radioactivity and affect any animals that eat it.

As expected, the earlier hay or silage is made following contamination with fall-out, the higher will be its radiation levels. Thus, following the fall-out from Chernobyl during the first week in May, the most contaminated hay had levels of up to 10,000 becquerels per kilogram. Once made, the winter feed would retain its radioactivity except for any lost through physical decay processes. For instance, hay made by the second week of June 1986 in the Drome region of France had a caesium content of 10,500 becquerels per kilogram according to measurements made a year later by CRII-RAD. A second cut of hay made in July 1986 showed levels of only 1,400 becquerels per kilogram. Nevertheless wide variations were found from one field to the next, depending on the precise patterns of rainfall, the fertility of the soil, and the time of cutting the crop.

Cattle consume the equivalent of 12 kilograms (26 pounds) of hay a day as winter feed. Therefore, if they were fed on the most contaminated hay, they could have ingested up to 120,000 becquerels of radioactive caesium each day. But how much of that caesium would actually get into meat?

An animal's body gradually eliminates caesium, taking approximately three months to get rid of half the amount present. The kidneys are the organs most highly contaminated with caesium. But if strontium is present, it resembles calcium and tends to accumulate in the bones and teeth, where it remains fixed for much of the life of the animal.

Taking a sheep or a goat as an example, on the basis that hay contains 6,000 becquerels of caesium per kilogram and the animal eats 2 kilograms a day, its daily intake is 12,000 becquerels. Approximately half of this gets excreted in the faeces and urine (leading to re-contamination of the pasture), and if the animal is milked up to 2,000 becquerels pass out in the milk (and can find their way into dairy products). In the animal itself, 540 becquerels pass into the meat, giving a concentration of about 18 becquerels per kilogram (8 becquerels per pound). In addition, 2,000 becquerels go into the kidneys and 1,000 becquerels into the liver.

The level of radioactivity to be found in animals depends on how they live. Game animals tend to survive in marginal wilderness areas away from rich farm land. As a result, after radioactive fall-out they accumulate relatively high levels of radiation compared to domesticated livestock, either kept indoors or fed on lush pastures.

The Institute for Research on Energy and Environment in Heidelberg, West Germany, made a study of the transfer of radioactivity from contaminated winter feed in southern Germany into milk and meat consumed by people in Bavaria and Baden-Wurttemberg. It indicated that the total collective effective dose to human beings from just that one source is likely to be in the region of 26,000 person-sieverts. This figure contrasts strongly with the number calculated by the United Kingdom National Radiological Protection Board for the collective dose for the entire West German population during 1986 of 14,000 person-sieverts, and for all time of 30,000 person-sieverts. According to the Heidelberg Institute, the effective dose from only the contaminated winter feed can be expected to lead to as many as 4,000 extra cancer cases – four times more than the total for the whole of the Common Market countries calculated over all time by the NRPB. The substantial differences in the numbers results from a different estimate of the dose and from a radically different assessment of its effects.

Until November 1987, the norms prevailing in much of the Common Market for permissible levels of contamination in food were 370 becquerels per kilogram for milk, dairy products and foodstuffs destined for babies, and 600 becquerels per kilogram for other foods. With these norms in mind, CRII-RAD found that at the end of 1986 in the French Drome and L'Ardeche regions which had received the highest fall-out, some 2 per cent of the meat from cattle exceeded 600 becquerels per kilogram. For sheep meat in the same districts, the percentage in excess of 600 becquerels per kilogram was 7, with some readings over 1,000 becquerels per kilogram. In France there were no restrictions against the sale of such meat.

In Britain, the limits for contamination of meat were set at 1,000 becquerels per kilogram. In the most contaminated areas in North Wales, Cumbria in England and parts of Scotland more than 100,000 animals remained with excess levels during 1986 and some 50,000 animals in 1987. The ban on the sale and consumption of the affected animals remained rigorously in force.

Because wild vegetation tends to be more efficient at concentrating radioactive material than well-fertilized domestic crops, game animals that live on wild plants are also likely to have higher levels of radioactivity compared with domestic ones. Reindeer have undoubtedly received the most publicity, and levels of caesium in some animals in northern Sweden exceeded 40,000 becquerels per kilogram by early February 1987. Whereas in Sweden the general level set for a ban on consumption of meat products was put at 300 becquerels per kilogram, in Norway the level was set at up to 20 times that level to help the Sami people whose livelihood depends on a viable market for reindeer products. Reindeer are particularly at risk because much of their diet comes from lichens, which retain absorbed radioactive isotopes.

Other wild animals are somewhat less at risk, but nonetheless more so than domestic animals. Analyses of the levels of radioactivity in woodcock made by the French National Office of Hunting revealed that 13 per cent of the birds studied had levels above 600 becquerels per kilogram in October 1986; 5 per cent in November; and 4 per cent in December. One bird was found with 5,000 becquerels per kilogram.

In November 1987 new norms for radioactive contamination were introduced into the Common Market countries. The acceptable levels were virtually doubled, with caesium levels in meat and other foodstuffs put at 1,250 becquerels per kilogram and in milk and dairy products at 1,000 becquerels per kilogram. For iodine-131 and strontium-90, the levels in foodstuffs other than milk were put at 3,000 becquerels per kilogram, and for milk and other dairy products at 500 becquerels per kilogram. As some critics commented, the new norms appear to have been arrived at in the acceptance that Chernobyl will be only the first of many major accidents in nuclear reactors in the years to come.

In Sweden one woodcock was discovered with 17,000 becquerels per kilogram in July 1986. Other game animals in Sweden were also found to have high radiation levels: hares, for instance, with 5,000 becquerels per kilogram; deer with 8,000; and elk with 1,000. The National Institute of Radiation Protection recommended that woodcock should not be hunted while the caesium levels remained high. No restrictions were imposed on hunting other game animals. In West Germany, near Lake Constance, one deer was found with 300,000 becquerels per kilogram in the thyroid.

﹏﹏ Fish ﹏﹏

Run-off is ultimately carried into rivers and lakes, where if it is radioactive it will contaminate fish and other aquatic animals. After Chernobyl, the first measurements of gamma activity in the lakes of regions with high fall-out during heavy rain gave readings of between 2,000 and 6,000 becquerels per litre, compared to some 15 becquerels per litre before the accident. In Scandinavia, by early autumn 1986 contamination in fish had gone up to levels of around 1,400 becquerels per kilogram. In winter the levels are likely to increase still further.

The uptake of iodine-131 in fish after the fall-out was surprisingly rapid. Fish in the Lake Constance region of West Germany were found with levels of the isotope as high as 5,400 becquerels per kilogram, which far exceeded the restrictions prevailing in West Germany that meat and fish with more than 200 becquerels per kilogram should be banned from consumption. In France, meanwhile, the permissible level of iodine-131 allowed in the flesh of animals was 8,000 becquerels per kilogram.

Radioactivity in fish: rain washes away radioactive fall-out, carrying it down slopes and into rivers and lakes. Fish take in radioactive substances from water, accumulating them in their flesh and other organs.

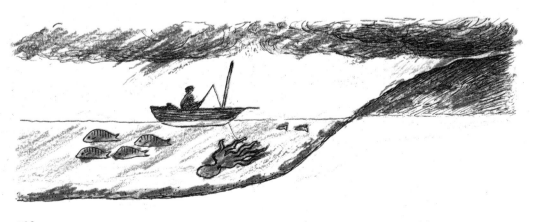

108

The authorities around Lake Constance were particularly enlightened about the consequences of radioactive contamination, and the public was swiftly informed that foodstuffs were likely to have high radiation levels. Despite the heavy fall-out in the region, at least on the West German side of the border it would seem that actual doses to the thyroid did not exceed 0.5 millisieverts in adults and 0.3 millisieverts in young children.

⁓⁓ Vegetables ⁓⁓

Once radioactive fall-out is deposited, large amounts are picked up by vegetables – particularly leafy ones such as lettuce and spinach. But after the fall-out has gone into the soil or decayed somewhat, contamination of such plants falls dramatically. You should therefore be very careful about eating vegetables in the first few months after fall-out, but you need not be so cautious later. Most green vegetables have a strong ability to take up radioactive iodine from the air.

In the first couple of weeks of May 1986, the University of Constance found that in the Lake Constance region a wide range of vegetables had radioactivity that was ten or more times higher than the limit of 250 becquerels per kilogram then prevailing in West Germany. Some of the specific readings were as follows: parsley had an average value of 2,900 becquerels per kilogram, with peaks of up to 5,900; spinach averaged 1,400 becquerels per kilogram, with peaks of 4,500; the average value for lettuce was 650 becquerels per kilogram, peaking at 7,200; radishes averaged 110 becquerels per kilogram, with peaks of 660; rhubarb had average values of 100 becquerels per kilogram, with a maximum of 320; and kohl rabi had values consistently below 160 becquerels per kilogram.

Washing vegetables removes only a few per cent of radioactivity at best, and even after cooking more than half of the original radioactivity is left in the leaves. Such a strong absorption of iodine-131 suggests that the radio-isotope is taken up quickly into the leaves through the respiratory pores (stomata) while the plant is in a phase of rapid growth, as in early summer. At the same time, both through physical decay and because of the rapid growth of the plant, the actual iodine content falls rapidly – a half-life of 2-3 days being observed. The local government put a ban on the consumption of such vegetables for nearly three weeks after fall-out had hit the Lake Constance region, and the vegetables were ploughed back into the soil.

Once iodine-131 levels have fallen, the main risk of contamination comes from caesium isotopes and to a much lesser extent from strontium-90 (present at about one-fiftieth of the caesium levels). Caesium competes with potassium for take-up by living organisms, including plants. Potassium does have its own radio-isotope – potassium-40 – and natural levels of radio-potassium in vegetables are around 100 becquerels per kilogram and in milk about 40 becquerels per litre. In the Lake Constance region, although levels of caesium fall-out had been high (typically 8,000 to 12,000 becquerels per square metre of ground), the uptake into vegetables was low. Levels also tended to fall even lower as the season progressed.

In general, vegetables and fruits tend to fall into two categories as regards uptake of caesium. At the lower end of the range with caesium contamina-

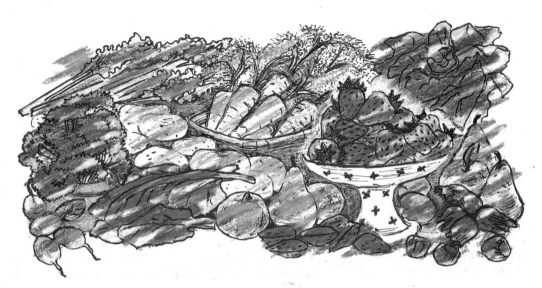

tion less than 30 becquerels per kilogram are the common European vegetables, apples, pears and cereals such as wheat and oats. In the higher range, with contamination levels of up to 100 becquerels per kilogram, are soft and stone fruits, rye, barley and winter feed for animals based on grass and herbal leys.

The degree to which caesium is able to get into plants depends very much on the nature of the soil. On a clay or loamy soil, it tends to be locked away in the soil structure and is less available for absorption by plants. But where the soils are lacking in minerals, the caesium remains far more available and higher contamination of plants can be expected. Measurements made by CRII-RAD in France in 1986 and 1987 very much mirrored the findings in southern West Germany, and regarding caesium contamination of vegetables, fruits, grains and plants in general a definite pattern emerges. This can be summarized as follows.

Garden vegetables are likely to have tens of becquerels of caesium per kilogram at most, the average values being below 30 during 1986 and dropping to half or less a year later. Most grains have similar values as vegetables, as do some common fruits (such as pears).

Nuts and fruits such as almonds, hazel nuts and apricots can have values that reach 300 becquerels per kilogram, whereas olives and grapes seem to have relatively low values in the region of 10 becquerels per kilogram.

Broad-leaved vegetables, such as lettuce and spinach, will pick up radioactive fall-out that has been deposited on them. Trees bearing nuts, such as almonds, are also efficient in taking in radioactive substances, this time from the soil. The richer the horticultural land the less radioactive isotopes get absorbed into the plant.

~~~~ Aromatic plants ~~~~

Aromatic plants do not merely supply herbs and spices to flavour food. On poorer soils, as for instance in the hills of the Mediterranean, they provide essential forage for the herds and flocks of farmers and shepherds. One year after Chernobyl the independent CRII-RAD laboratory had carried out more than 200 analyses of aromatic plants of different species and from

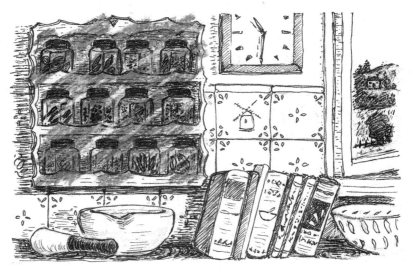

Many herbs, such as thyme and rosemary, thrive on barren, rocky slopes up in the Mediterranian mountains. They are particularly proficient in concentrating radioactive fall-out.

different regions in France. In essence, it found that the sooner the plants had been cut or picked after fall-out, the more contaminated they were. Nevertheless, the greatest variation in the levels of radioactivity lay in the variation in species. Ordinary thyme headed the list – the highest concentration actually measured being of the order of more than 26,000 becquerels per kilogram. The highest level in sage in comparison was 620 becquerels per kilogram.

In general, aromatic plants live on soils that are low in minerals, with the result that they are quick to take in radioactive elements such as ruthenium, strontium, caesium and iodine-131. Because the soils are poorer and do not receive artificial fertilization, wild-growing herbs tend to concentrate radioactive fall-out more heavily than do cultivated herbs.

Herbs such thyme, rosemary and serpolet, which are adapted to semi-arid conditions, have abundant leaves for absorbing moisture from the air, in particular dew, and have an extensive root system. Moreover such plants open up their leaves during rainfall, and should the rain be rich in fall-out, as it was in the first week in May, the radioactive minerals would be swiftly absorbed and carried to the interior of the leafy material. At best, washing the picked plants shortly after the rains even with soft detergents would wash out no more than 20 per cent of the radioactivity which had fallen onto them. Most of such plants have a particular propensity for picking up caesium, which sufficiently resembles potassium. Thyme especially contains a binding substance which holds any minerals that have landed on the leaves until they can be absorbed. Lichens too have similar properties.

Nonetheless, if the aromatic herb is not cut early after the fall-out but a month or more later, the radioactivity is found to have fallen by an amount which depends on both the physical half-life of the radioactive element concerned and on the time taken to eliminate that substance from the plant's tissues. The two caesiums, 134 and 137, have an effective half-life in the plant of around 13 days, whereas for another important radionuclide, ruthenium-103 (which has a physical half-life of just 39 days), the effective half-life is 11 days.

Herbs such as thyme absorb radioactive substances from the air. On poor soils radioactive caesium stays mobile and is quickly taken up by the plant. On better soils radioactive caesium tends to get locked away in the soil and is far less available. But even on good soils herbs, being more efficient at concentrating radioactive fall-out especially from the air, are still more likely to be contaminated than root crops such as carrots.

However, after being eliminated from the plant, such minerals pass into the surface of the soil and can get re-suspended. They can then be incorporated anew. As a result, the contamination of aromatic plants appears to go in waves, but all the time with the overall levels decreasing. This pattern of contamination, elimination to the soil and recontamination appears to be what happened on poor pastureland in the fall-out contaminated areas of Britain, resulting in subsequent high levels of caesium in sheep.

Studies carried out by CRII-RAD show that the soil under an aromatic herb is five times more contaminated with radioactive minerals compared with soil several metres away and bearing no plants. Moreover most of the radioactive minerals are found within a centimetre below the soil surface. The opportunites for the recontamination of the plant are very high.

The quantities of aromatic plants used in a country such as France, for both cookery and perfumes, are considerable. In fact, French people consume 23,000 tonnes of a variety of herbs each year. About 8,000 tonnes are local produce and 20,000 tonnes are imported. The difference of 5,000 tonnes are exported from France, mostly to other countries of the Common Market.

Certain of the herbs are used as medicinal plants and pharmaceutical products. Whereas in France no control at all was imposed on the use of medicinal herbs in pharmaceutical preparations following Chernobyl, in neighbouring Switzerland the ruling was that the same norms should prevail as had been laid down for foods – namely that the concentrations of caesium-137 and caesium-134 should not exceed 600 becquerels per kilogram.

Mushrooms

Remarkably high levels of radioactive contamination can build up in mushrooms, and unless you know exactly where they come from (particularly some of the more exotic edible species) it is best to limit consumption to a kilogram or less per week. With regard to long-lived radio-isotopes such as caesium-137, mushrooms appear to retain the activity over many years.

Radioactivity in mushrooms: some species of wild mushrooms are very efficient in taking up radioactive substances such as caesium-137 from the soil, and concentrations can become very high.

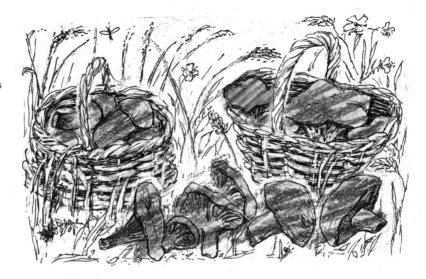

Measurements made by CRII-RAD from the areas of Aveyron, Loire and Haute-Loire in France indicated high radiation levels in mushrooms that had been picked even before the Chernobyl incident. Some chanterelles from the Loire that had been picked in October 1985 gave readings as high as 8,500 becquerels per kilogram. The source of those high readings must have been fall-out from the atmospheric nuclear tests of the 1960s, and it was indicative that caesium-134, the shorter-lived isotope of the element, was present in very low quantities of only 20 becquerels per kilogram.

Mushrooms vary considerably in the amount of caesium they absorb from the soil. According to CRII-RAD, the most contaminated were *Boletus chrysenteron*, with 24,500 becquerels per kilogram; *Lactarius plombeus*, with 18,900; *Boletus badius*, with 15,460; *Laccaria amethystae*, with 15,120; *Cantarellus tubiformis*, with 9,115; *Hydnum repandum* and *Boletus elegans*, with around 3,000; and *Craterellus cornucopioides*, with 1,840 becquerels per kilogram.

All these high levels were found in regions of France that had been most affected by Chernobyl fall-out, and the ratio of caesium-134 to caesium-137 indicated that the contamination was of recent origin. The measurements were of dry matter, and therefore indicated a higher concentration than would be found in fresh mushrooms. The Common Market norm of 600 becquerels per kilogram of fresh vegetable material corresponds to some 6,000 becquerels of dry matter. The concentrations found in many of the species of mushrooms collected in the high fall-out areas therefore exceeds the norms established by the EEC after Chernobyl.

It seems that many species of mushrooms will continue to build up and retain high levels of caesium in the the years to come. In that respect, mushrooms behave like lichens and mosses.

Honey

Because honeybees forage over a wide range of plants, they can carry radioactively contaminated pollen and nectar into the hive. Moreover, because bees feed on the resulting honey, they are likely to retain a fairly high level of radioisotopes in their bodies. Various measurements made of bees, honey, pollen and beeswax following Chernobyl show that levels of caesium contamination can reach several hundred becquerels per kilogram.

It would appear that pollen is directly contaminated by fall-out rather than by transfer from other parts of the plant, whereas nectar is contaminated by the transfer of caesium as the nectar is being manufactured by the plant. Pollen is therefore unlikely to be contaminated two years running from the same fall-out, whereas nectar (a metabolic product) may still incorporate some caesium.

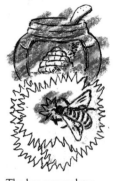

The bee accumulates radioactive fall-out by collecting pollen or nectar from flowers. Long-lived radioactive substances such as caesium tend therefore to get into the honey.

Rainwater

Fall-out is not only washed out of the plume by rain, but once on the ground tends to be carried either to surface waters or through the soil to groundwaters. For longer-lived radioactivity, such as that from caesium, radiation levels in bodies of water are therefore likely to increase with time over the course of the first year following a large radiation release. Where rainwater was heavily contaminated, as in North Wales in the first week of May 1986, the British government advised against drinking it. The NRPB has calculated the DERLs for drinking water on the basis that a one-year-old baby drinks up to 0.7 litres (1.2 pints) a day, a ten-year-old child 0.95 litres (1.7 pints), and an adult 1.65 litres (2.9 pints).

A decision to limit the drinking of contaminated supplies should be considered when the concentration of iodine-131 has reached 10,000 becquerels per litre, and certainly be in effect when it reaches 35,000 becquerels per litre. Similar orders of magnitude are indicated for caesium, strontium and ruthenium. The values are therefore close to those applied for a ban on drinking milk, and again the most restrictive group is taken to be one-year-old children. If a ban on drinking water is applied, alternative supplies have to be found.

Clearly, if you have time to put aside water for drinking before a radioactive plume is likely to pass overhead, then such a precaution is worth while. Even if the water is not needed, it is better to be prepared than be anxious about possible contamination at a later date.

✦✦✦ Measuring fall-out in food ✦✦✦

It is not only consumers in cities and towns who want to know how much radiation is in their food, farmers too are concerned about what may be in their produce. Governments basically can carry out spot checks but would be hard-pressed to respond to each individual request for testing. The Chernobyl accident spawned a number of independent testing laboratories, which set out to provide a service for those wanting to know radiation levels in foods and soils, and filled a yawning gap left by government laboratory services.

One of the most efficient and informative of the new laboratory services has been CRII-RAD – Commission Regionale Independent d'Information sur la Radioactivité – which set up in Montelimar, near Lyon in France. Within a few months of May 1986, CRII-RAD had carried out more than 500 measurements in different plants and food products from various regions in France, and were publishing the results in a quarterly magazine. The magazine – *Le Cri du Rad* – also contains comments on the significance of the results as well as some basic information about radiation and its possible effects.

In particular CRII-RAD found that certain kinds of products from certain regions in France remained highly contaminated with fall-out during 1986 and 1987. The highest activities were found in mountain herbs, especially thyme, and in mushrooms and in hay made at certain times of the year in contaminated areas such as Corsica.

In West Germany, an excellent service for measuring radiation in foodstuffs and the environment was established in Bremen. The institute, known as Arbeitsgemeinschaft ökologischer Forschingsinstitute (AGF) has been publishing monthly results following Chernobyl (see Appendix).

Caesium in milk and meat

Grass is far more effective at concentrating caesium fall-out than are most plants, and this characteristic is reflected in the high levels of caesium found in hay and silage made in 1986. In the Lake Constance region, grass cut in May 1986 had caesium levels averaging some 2,000 becquerels per kilogram, reaching peak levels of 4,000 becquerels. In Corsica and regions of France such as Drome, levels of caesium in hay from some fields exceeded 10,000 becquerels per kilogram.

Experiments carried out by the University of Constance on the transfer of caesium from contaminated feed into cow's milk and into the animal's flesh indicated that up to 4 per cent of the element taken into the body gets into the milk (giving some 50 becquerels per litre), with an equilibrium at that level being reached in one or two weeks. Some of the cows slaughtered after six weeks' feeding on contaminated hay and silage had up to 100 becquerels per kilogram in their meat.

The local government of Baden-Wurttemberg was concerned that the radiation dose of 30 millirems (0.3 millisieverts) should not be exceeded over the course of a year by members of the public, and in particular by young children with a high milk consumption. For this reason, the University set out to test whether judicious feeding of cows with a mixture of uncontaminated concentrates and hay and silage from a later cut in the year could reduce the average contamination level of milk to no more than 30 becquerels per litre. Experiments with cattle fed on nothing but uncontaminated feed showed that within 20 days the levels of caesium in milk could be reduced down to some 5 becquerels per litre.

Meanwhile, if a child of about a year old were to drink half a litre (nearly a pint) of milk each day contaminated with 30 becquerels per litre, the dose at the end of a year would be 0.35 millisieverts.

Radiation dose from caesium

During 1986 and 1987, the EEC norms for maximum recommended levels of caesium in foodstuffs stood at 370 becquerels per litre of milk and 600 becquerels per kilogram for all other foods. It has to be appreciated that if children consumed foods with caesium at those maximum permissible levels, during a year they would receive radiation doses practically double the 5 millisieverts maximum permissible level recommended by the International Commission on Radiological Protection.

115

In the event, except in foodstuffs such as nuts, mushrooms, certain dairy products and meat (especially game), even in the most contaminated areas of western Europe overall radiation doses could be kept down as long as certain sensible precautions were taken.

Taking into account consumption levels of common foodstuffs and the levels of contamination found in the Lake Constance region, scientists from the University estimated that the average dose over 1986 would be 0.2 millisievert, with much of the radiation coming from caesium in meat. Children, with a lower meat consumption than adults, would therefore be likely to receive lower doses still. On the other hand, a person who ate relatively large quantities of wild game, fish and mushrooms could receive up to 1 millisievert a year – approximately half as much again as the natural background radiation.

In fact, as the accident at Chernobyl underscored, the highest levels of radioactive contamination tend to be found in the more natural foods. Somebody who eats mainly these will unfortunately receive a larger radiation dose than the highly conventional modern person who lives basically off pre-packaged food which rather than originating locally is likely to come from almost anywhere in the world.

Another main group at risk are those farmers and their families who live in areas of relatively high fall-out and traditionally eat their own produce. In Sweden, several farmers were found to have a few thousand becquerels of caesium in their bodies, and relatively high levels have also been found in some people living in Cumbria and North Wales. Undoubtedly those with the highest levels in their bodies will be the Sami of northern Scandinavia who are at the top of a food chain that must rank as one of the most efficient in its ability to concentrate nuclear fall-out. The tragedy for the Sami is that a change in their eating habits and lifestyles signifies an end to traditional ways of life. Their own vulnerability to an accident that happened more than 1,000 kilometres (625 miles) away must certainly alert us to the appalling consequences of a major nuclear accident in the middle of crowded Europe, for instance just 50 kilometres (about 30 miles) from Paris or the same distance upwind from London.

Shelter

The social and economic cost of evacuating lots of people is very high, and the authorities naturally want to avoid such measures until they are convinced that the cost to health – physically and psychologically – would be even greater if the people were to remain behind. Most nuclear power stations are sited well away from large population centres, a prime concern being the difficulty of evacuating people in the event of a major radiation escape. Nonetheless, in a densely populated country it is virtually impossible to site a nuclear power station more than 30 or so kilometers (about 20 miles) away from any town or city. The declared aim is to reduce the likelihood of a Chernobyl-type disaster to such an extremely low level that the chances of it happening are virtually nil. And on that basis, in Britain the authorities plan for evacuating people only within a few kilometres of the plant. The Soviets meanwhile had to evacuate an area within a

If there is any chance that the radioactive plume is coming your way, bring in clothing off the line, shut all windows, switch off ventilation and go inside. If you need to go out for an urgent reason, do not bring the shoes that you have been wearing into the house. Leave them outside.

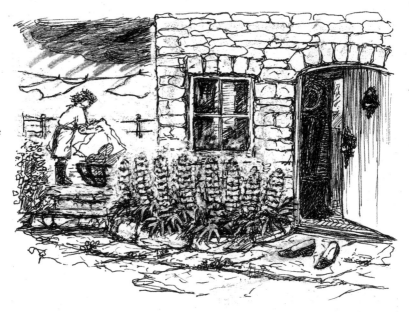

30-kilometre (19-mile) radius of Chernobyl, in addition to some communities much farther away.

In the event of an accident at a nearby nuclear power installation, it will be up to individual people as well as the authorities to decide whether evacuation is necessary. Nevertheless, until you can be satisfied beyond all reasonable doubt that the radiation release (if there has been one) is limited in extent, you should take shelter.

The obvious precautions include staying indoors with the windows firmly shut, at least while the plume is overhead, closing down any ventilation system, bringing in any washing hanging outside, getting in any domestic pets, sealing off any open fireplaces, and putting away carpets, rugs, curtains and clothing so that they remain as free from dust as possible.

It is also important to take plenty of baths or showers – at least once a day – and to avoid going outside unless absolutely necessary. Shoes worn outside (and possibly contaminated) should be left outside and not taken indoors. Children in particular should be kept away from playgrounds and sandpits.

If you have a vegetable garden and can cover it with a plastic sheet, then all to the good. In the meantime, you should avoid eating local produce until you are sure that the radioactive contamination level is minimal. You should also make sure that there is a stock of fresh, covered water, as well as food that has been bought in from areas that have remained clear of any fall-out. Alternatively, food already in the home should be covered and protected. Food in a refrigerator or freezer should be safe.

Clothes and bed linen should be washed every day. If you have to go out in the rain, cover as much as yourself as possible with completely waterproof clothing, including rubber boots. Cover your mouth and nose with a damp disposable cloth to prevent inhaling or swallowing any radioactive particles.

To be certain that food is free from contamination, it is best to avoid consuming any fresh milk or dairy products for at least 40 days, because that will give time for any radioactive iodine to decay to harmless levels. Meat should also be avoided until you know whether or not it is contaminated and to what level.

If possible avoid pregnancy while levels of contamination are high. If a woman is already pregnant when the nuclear accident happens and she may have become contaminated, it is worth seeking advice about any risks to the foetus. A radiation dose to the whole body (and therefore to the foetus) of 5 millisieverts is cause for concern – it is likely to double the childhood cancer rate. If the baby is already born and being breast-fed, it is best to continue feeding in this way as long as the mother avoids contamination herself. Only a small proportion of radioactive substances passes into the milk of humans.

Housing

The type of housing you live or work in can make a considerable difference to the degree of exposure to external gamma radiation. The least protection comes from a wooden, single-family dwelling, and the most protection from a concrete building such as a block of apartments or offices. A wooden or lightly-built structure screens about 50 per cent of the radiation from a passing plume or fall-out, whereas high-rise apartments or office blocks screen about 90 per cent. In Sweden, in areas such as Gävle which received the highest fall-out from Chernobyl, the Institute of Radiation Protection estimated that somebody spending eight hours out of doors and the rest of the day in a family dwelling made of wood received a radiation dose of about 4 millisieverts during 1986, falling to 3 millisieverts through 1987 from external radiation as well as through breathing. If only two hours were spent outside rather than eight, the total radiation dose fell by a quarter. Meanwhile somebody who was in an office block or an apartment building probably received 2.4 millisieverts effective dose during 1986 if eight hours were spent outdoors and only 1.1 millisieverts if only two hours were spent outside. The average background radiation dose (see chapter 2) is 2 millisieverts a year.

The Derived Emergency Reference Level (DERL) for advising that shelter should be taken is defined as about 1,700 million becquerels for each second in each cubic metre of air for a radioisotope such as caesium-137. By the time radiation has reached five times that level, shelter should already have been taken, according to the British National Radiological Protection Board. The DERLs for radioactive actinides such as plutonium-239 are considerably lower at less than a million becquerels per second per cubic metre of air. For iodine-131, the DERL is approximately five times lower than for caesium-137, because the critical group person is taken to be a 10-year-old child, whose thyroid gland is particularly at risk.

At most, sheltering can be continued for only a few days, and should fall-out levels be high enough to make it risky to spend more than a very short time outside, it is clearly best to move away. One problem, of course, is that unless you are officially advised to leave the area, it will be difficult later to obtain compensation for abandoning your home and your work. For this reason, it is important to have independent monitoring of the radiation levels in a contaminated area, carried out by scientists who can properly

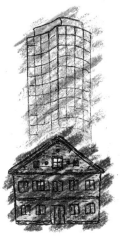

Some buildings are more effective in shielding us from radiation than are others. The best protection is found in high rise, concrete office blocks or apartments. The least from traditional wooden structures.

interpret the results. That way you can at least be reassured that taking shelter for a few days or even hours will give adequate protection.

Nevertheless, even when it is considered safe to go out and resume a more normal existence, you should remain out of doors for as little as possible during the first weeks after the passage of the plume (to allow all the shorter-lived radionuclides to decay to harmless levels).

Children's play areas

After the Chernobyl accident, outdoor sandboxes of kindergartens in the Munich area showed average contamination levels that at nearly 50,000 becquerels per square metre were some 40 times higher than previously. Some sandboxes had nearly 110,000 becquerels per square metre. An independent physicist, Xaver Brenner, from the Umwelt Institut pointed out that the radiation was not evenly spread but concentrated in particle hot spots which, if breathed into the lungs of a child or swallowed, would give extremely high localized radiation doses. Clearly, in the event of a nuclear accident, it is essential that all contaminated sand be removed from such play areas and replaced by uncontaminated sand.

Filtered air

Modern buildings with air-conditioning take in air through filters. In the event of radioactive fall-out, the filters become highly contaminated. They should therefore be serviced following an accident by people properly trained in dealing with radioactivity. Motor vehicles also use air filters to clean out dust particles, and in areas that have received high levels of fall-out not only will the surface of the vehicle be coated but the filters will concentrate radioactive particles. Servicing such vehicles should not therefore be left to ordinary garage mechanics. The filters themselves will also need to be disposed of in a safe way.

Rain

If it rains when a radioactive plume is passing overhead, the immediate danger (as we have seen for Chernobyl) from radioactive aerosols and particles in the air is far outweighed by the deposition of radioactive substances on buildings and on the ground. Radioisotopes such as those of caesium are readily washed out with rain, and even though initially there was ten times less caesium in the Chernobyl plume compared with iodine-131, in some places (such as Britain) the amounts of the two elements deposited during a rainstorm wash-out were similar. Thus in areas where it was dry while the plume was passing, there was ten times less caesium deposition on the ground than iodine.

The highest levels of fall-out are bound to occur close to the site of the accident, particularly of less volatile particles such as those made up of actinides and other alpha-emitters. Even after thorough clean-up operations, it is likely to be decades before people can safely move back into an evacuated area such as that near Chernobyl.

Decontamination is an extremely costly process involving an attempt to collect as much as possible of the fall-out. The Soviets sprayed a light, sticky plastic film over the surface of the ground, which was later gathered up and disposed of. The first few centimetres of topsoil also have to be taken away and disposed of in a secure landfill site. Coating buildings with a special paint and tarring roads are other ways of binding radioactive fall-out for subsequent collection and disposal. In the immediate aftermath of the Chernobyl accident, the Soviets were seen hosing down vehicles, roads and buildings. According to experts in the United States, such action is ill-advised because it disperses the radioactive debris into the soil and ground-water, thus exposing populations farther afield. The main task after a major radiation release should be to confine the contamination and dispose of it at a safe site.

Farms

Nuclear installations are generally sited in the countryside, and inevitably farmland gets contaminated with fall-out after an accident. If the fall-out is heavy, it may be thought necessary to remove a few centimetres of topsoil and then plough the land deeply to carry radionuclides sufficiently beneath the surface to reduce ground gamma radiation and lessen the chances of shallow-rooted plants picking up radiation.

Before the Chernobyl disaster it was known that clay soils were far more effective at binding radionuclides such as caesium than are soils rich in organic matter, such as the acid, peaty soils found in hilly areas overlying granite. What did prove surprising following Chernobyl was the extent to which caesium fall-out remained available for uptake into plants and therefore into grazing animals such as sheep and cattle.

Some radionuclides are far more readily taken into plants than others. Iodine is quickly absorbed, and within two days finds its way into the milk of grazing animals. The rates of absorption of caesium and strontium are somewhat slower, taking about a week. On the other hand, radio-iodine will have decayed by some 15 per cent in the two days it takes to get into milk, whereas the activity of both caesium-137 and strontium-90 is hardly diminished by a week's delay.

The uptake by plants of actinides such as plutonium and americium, should they be present in fall-out, is far lower. But they are dangerous because they are easily blown around and re-suspended in the air, from which they can be breathed in. If actinides get carried into coastal waters or into lakes, bottom-dwelling animals and certain species of bacteria concentrate them so that they get taken into the food chain. Indeed, actinides discharged into the Irish Sea from the Sellafield reprocessing works in Cumbria appear to have come back ashore through a combination of various mechanisms, including concentration in bottom-dwelling creatures and through forming aerosols, possibly with the aid of micro-organisms.

Just as the thyroid gland can be protected from radioactive iodine by ensuring that it has already been stocked up with stable iodine, so is it possible to some extent to prevent the uptake of caesium into crops by fertilizing the ground with potash or other fertilizers rich in potassium. The poorer the soils, as are those in Lapland and in the uplands of North Wales and Cumbria, the more readily is caesium available for uptake.

At least during the early stages after a nuclear accident, and while the plume is known to be in the vicinity, farmers should keep their livestock under cover and provide them with feed that has not been contaminated. In

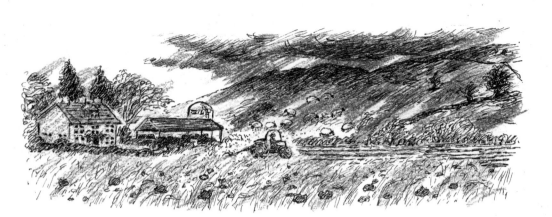

Because it tends to rain more in the uplands, washing out atmospheric pollutants, and because the soil is poorer, radioactive fall-out tends to accumulate in vegetation and in grazing animals up in the hills. Low lying areas, with richer soils and lower rainfall gather less fall-out.

the Netherlands, parts of West Germany and the most heavily affected areas of Sweden, farmers were advised to keep their cattle under cover until they were told it was safe to let them out. Dutch farmers who disobeyed such orders were fined. In much of northern Europe and indeed in the United States, the housing of animals during winter does not present any problems because that is how they are usually kept anyway. The problem arises in the late spring, summer or autumn, when the animals are traditionally outside. In spring there may be little or no winter feed left, and in autumn no farmer would want to use up the reserves of silage and hay put by for the winter. Moreover, spring is the time when grass is growing at its best and most nutritious, and few farmers would want to forego that time of the year for grazing their animals.

Be aware

In the event, in highly contaminated areas, decisions have to made whether to move livestock elsewhere or, if that proves impossible, to slaughter them for human consumption before they become contaminated.

As we have learned, we cannot detect radiation with our senses. We have to rely on instruments to tell us where radiation is and how much there is of it. Before the accident at Chernobyl, government authorities had virtually the only facilities for carrying out radiation monitoring. In general they had a vested interest in supporting the nuclear industry and, if anything, there was a tendency to underplay the consequences of any accidents. Today there are a number of independent monitoring bodies that can provide information about radiation levels, enabling individuals to come to responsible decisions. And once we know what the radiation levels are in foodstuffs and in our immediate environment, we can take action to lessen the risks to ourselves and our families. Awareness is the key.

CHAPTER

⚜ 6 ⚜

Introduction to the food tables

⚜ Radioactive contamination in food and drink ⚜

This chapter sets out to provide essential information about the levels of radioactive contamination that can be expected in various foodstuffs after fall-out from a nuclear accident. The values given have been calculated using broad generalizations, based on current models of the pattern of fall-out and the movements of radioactive substances through the food chain and into our bodies.

After a nuclear accident, the levels of fall-out vary enormously from place to place, and it would therefore be impractical to map out every possible variation in contamination. Instead information is given for two situations: a high level of fall-out, as might occur when heavy rain has washed through the radioactive plume, and a much lower level of fall-out, as would be deposited on the ground by a similar plume during dry weather. Both of these phenomena – plume-washed radioactivity and dry deposition – were observed after the Chernobyl accident. Not only were the levels of fall-out strikingly different, but so too were the proportions of the two most significant radio-isotopes, iodine-131 and caesium-137.

In the following tables and charts, reference is made to just three elements: radio-iodine (iodine-131), caesium (both isotopes, 134 and 137) and strontium (strontium-90). These are chosen because, in general, they are likely to be the most significant following a nuclear accident. Many other radio-isotopes, including plutonium, also escape, but usually in far less significant quantities.

The levels of fall-out chosen for the tables are based on a relationship between the three elements that was observed in many places after Chernobyl. As much as 15 times more iodine-131 was deposited on the ground after heavy rain than through dry fall-out. If therefore 200,000 becquerels per square metre of radio-iodine is taken as the amount falling out after heavy rain has washed through the plume, the dry deposition will be 13,000 becquerels per square metre.

Under dry conditions, some five times less caesium is likely to be deposited on average compared with iodine-131. The value for caesium fall-out is therefore 2,600 becquerels per square metre of ground. On the other hand, because caesium is less volatile than iodine, whenever it rains heavily through the plume proportionately greater quantities may be deposited than under dry conditions. The levels of caesium may even come close to matching those of iodine. Therefore, in our scenario, we have assumed that as much as 200,000 becquerels per square metre of caesium has fallen out.

Strontium-90 contributes least to overall radioactive contamination, being present at approximately 2 per cent of the caesium levels. This is equivalent to some 4,000 becquerels per square metre under wet conditions, and 40 becquerels per square metre under dry conditions.

Radioactivity in cow's milk

On average pasture, a quarter of the iodine, caesium and strontium deposited is incorporated into the grass. A cow consumes the grass from approximately 100 square metres of pasture each day. It is therefore possible to estimate the total quantity of each radionuclide taken into the cow – and then into its milk. It should be appreciated that the levels indicated are those that would occur if cattle are grazing the pasture while or shortly after the deposition happens. By keeping the cows off the pasture and under cover, farmers can largely avoid such high levels of contamination in milk (particularly of radio-iodine). The tables show what could happen in terms of radioactive contamination if no such precautions are taken.

The radiation dose

Natural radioactive decay and weathering in the soil gradually reduce the levels of radio-isotopes in pasture, and the radiation doses consequently fall. The information given on the doses incurred through consuming milk and dairy products is therefore based on the assumption that little or no advice is given or any bans placed on the actual food products themselves.

It has been found that both goat's milk and sheep's milk become far more contaminated than cow's milk, as do their dairy products. The levels of radioactive contamination in other foodstuffs, including meat, vegetables and drinks, vary considerably, but in general they are less than those found in milk and dairy products.

After the food charts, there are some typical menus, where radiation doses have been calculated on the assumption that the various items are eaten regularly every day. For instance, if an adult eats each day one omelette made with cow's milk, wild mushrooms and herbs from a highly contaminated wet-deposition region, the overall dose over a year will be 2 millisieverts. This is equal to the average natural background dose and just under half the ICRP's maximum recommended dose.

An infant, on the other hand, eating a smaller portion, will receive the much higher dose of 12 millisieverts. The substantial difference results from an infant's far greater sensitivity to radioactive contamination. Nevertheless, by far the greatest proportion of the dose comes from milk and dairy products. Indeed, it becomes clear that if we wish to limit radiation doses to ourselves following radioactive fall-out, we should only consume dairy products in sparing quantities – especially milk, yoghurt and cheeses – until we know that the radiation levels in them are acceptably low (and well below the norms recommended by the EEC). As before, the assumption remains that no bans or restrictions are placed on either the producer of the food or the consumer.

One lesson to be learned from the food charts and tables is that the more wholesome a food product is, and the more it has been produced under natural conditions, the more likely it is to become heavily contaminated with radioactivity following a nuclear accident. Wild edible mushrooms, wild game, goat's and sheep's cheeses, fish from mountain lakes, wild herbs, nuts, fruit, and honey – these are the risky foods after fall-out. In terms of radioactivity, the safe foods are those processed and preserved before the accident occurred, as well as those derived from low fall-out regions with good agricultural soils.

The tables can also be used to give an idea of the likely contamination for other levels of fall-out. Whatever fraction they are of the deposition levels in the tables, they will be reflected as an equivalent fraction of the radiation levels in the various foodstuffs, and finally of the radiation doses. The tables therefore also offer some flexibility in making up menus and diets in terms of probable radiation levels.

The following tables (pages 125–131) show what the levels of radioactive contamination in food products are likely to be, as a result of particular levels of deposition on the ground of iodine, caesium and, when relevant, strontium. Two levels of deposition are used for each radionuclide – one under dry conditions, the other under wet ones. The square under each of the food products is shaded according to the extent to which the level of contamination is a proportion of the relevant norms now in force in the EEC (see Appendix page 150). To cover the wide range of contamination that is likely to be encountered in different foodstuffs, each square when fully shaded represents ten times the EEC limit. A strip of shading in the square is therefore equivalent to the EEC norm. When a square has a radioactive hazard sign, the norm has been exceeded by at least fifty times. A tick represents minimal contamination.

These tables demonstrate the substantial differences in levels of contamination between fall-out under dry and wet conditions. They also show that dairy products under both conditions are likely to have unacceptable levels of contamination, particularly for iodine-131, and to a lesser extent for caesium. It should be stressed that such high levels result when the animals are out and grazing on pasture when the deposition occurs and are allowed to continue grazing. In fact, over the first month following deposition, iodine-131 levels in all foodstuffs fall substantially because of the natural decay of the radio-isotope and because of weathering. Both caesium and strontium are likely to be longer-term contaminants.

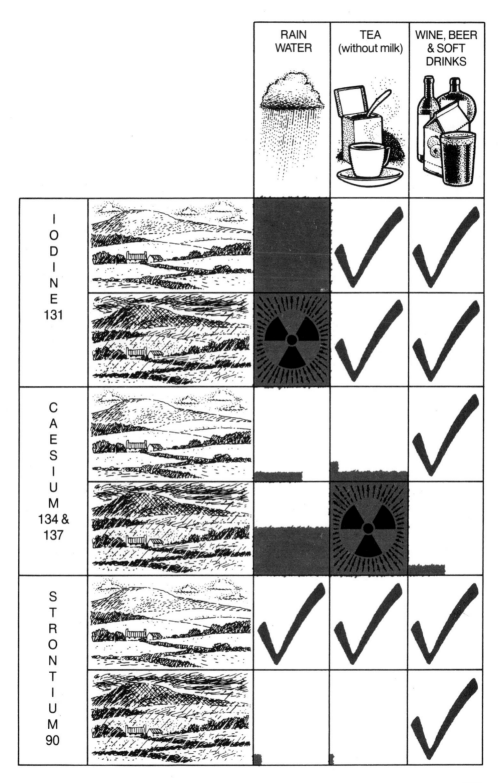

		RAIN WATER	TEA (without milk)	WINE, BEER & SOFT DRINKS
IODINE 131			✓	✓
		☢	✓	✓
CAESIUM 134 & 137				✓
			☢	
STRONTIUM 90		✓	✓	✓
				✓

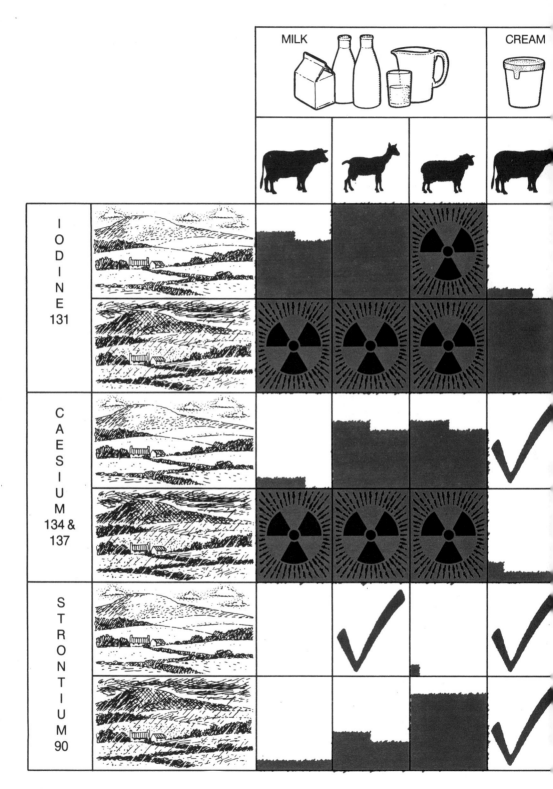

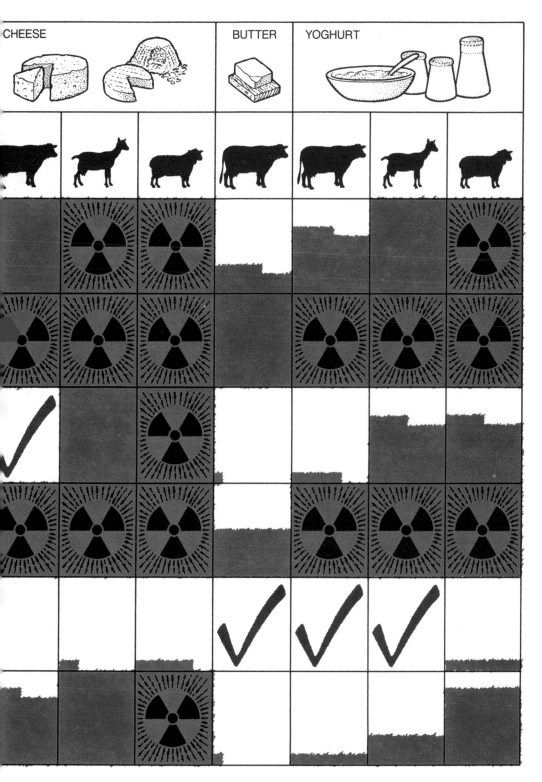

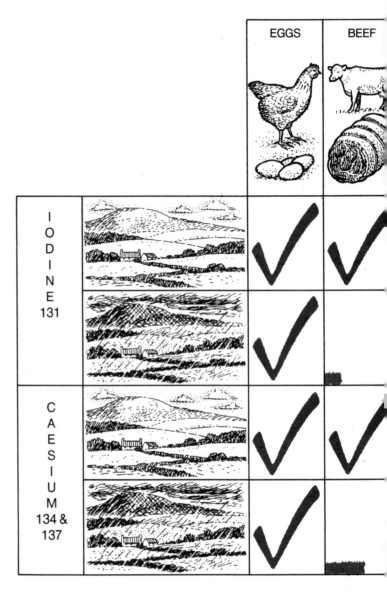

		EGGS	BEEF
I O D I N E 131		✓	✓
		✓	
C A E S I U M 134 & 137		✓	✓
		✓	

LAMB	PORK	CHICKEN	GAME	FISH (fresh-water)	FISH (sea-water)	SHELLFISH

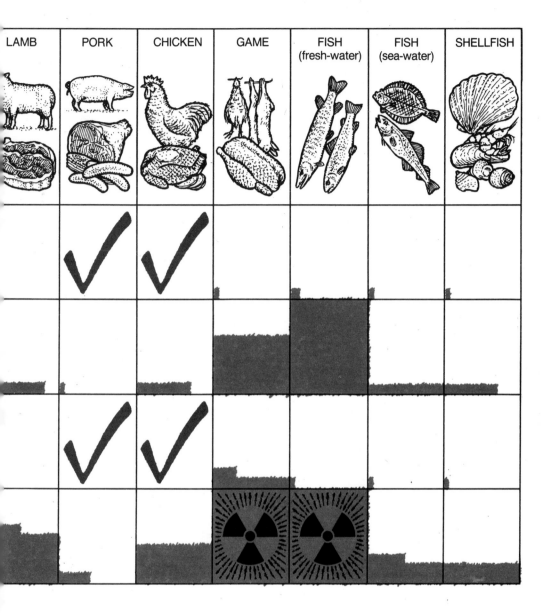

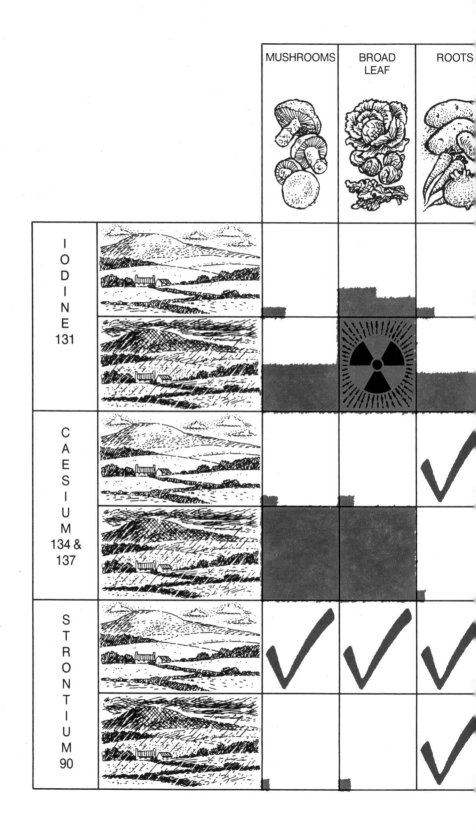

		MUSHROOMS	BROAD LEAF	ROOTS
I O D I N E 131				
C A E S I U M 134 & 137				✓
S T R O N T I U M 90		✓	✓	✓

GRAINS	HERBS	NUTS	SOFT FRUIT	APPLES & PEARS	STONED FRUIT	HONEY
✓		✓		✓		✓
✓		✓				✓
✓		✓	✓	✓	✓	✓
✓	✓	✓	✓	✓	✓	✓
✓		✓	✓	✓		✓

The following tables (pages 132–138) show the likely radiation doses that would accrue to infants, 10-year-old children and adults if they consumed foodstuffs in the quantities given on a daily basis. The doses are estimated on the assumption that no bans or restrictions are put on the production and harvesting of food. The doses are thus the consequences of continuing to consume food that is taken from areas contaminated by fall-out. They are therefore accumulated doses, taking account of the natural processes of radioactive decay in the environment. As a general rule the one-off dose acquired through consuming the food products for the one day following initial contamination by fall-out will be one-tenth of the accumulated dose.

The doses for infants are based on the assumption that they consume half the adult quantity of foodstuffs.

• Each square represents one millisievert of dose – a dose level that is considered the maximum a person should receive on a regular yearly basis. A dose above 50 millisievert is indicated by a radioactive hazard sign.

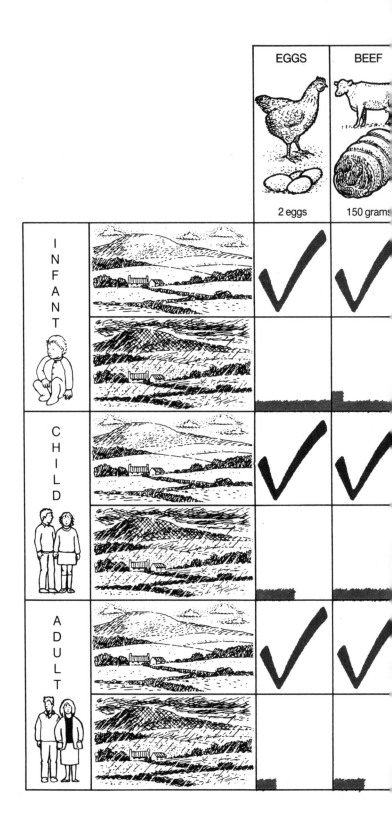

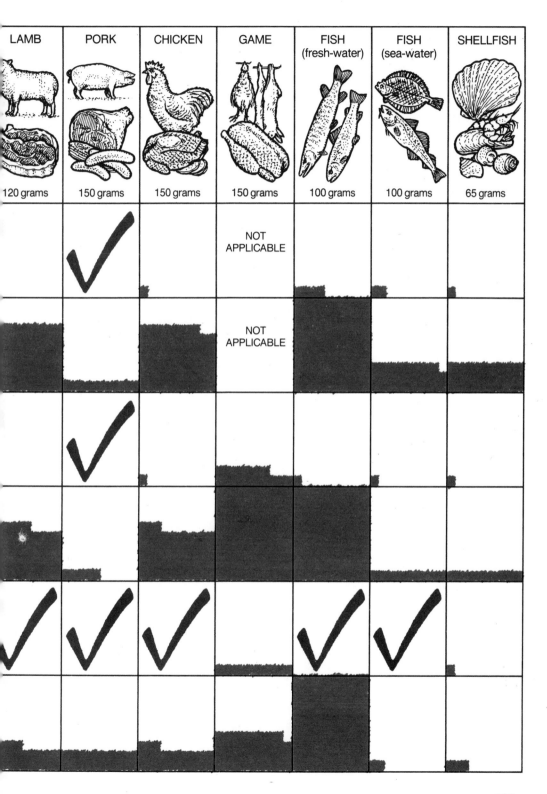

LAMB	PORK	CHICKEN	GAME	FISH (fresh-water)	FISH (sea-water)	SHELLFISH
120 grams	150 grams	150 grams	150 grams	100 grams	100 grams	65 grams
	✓		NOT APPLICABLE			
			NOT APPLICABLE			
	✓					
✓	✓	✓		✓	✓	

133

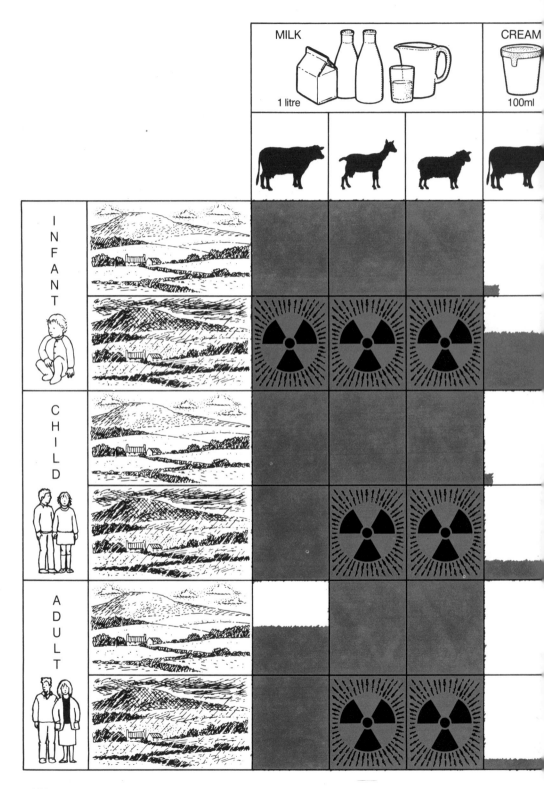

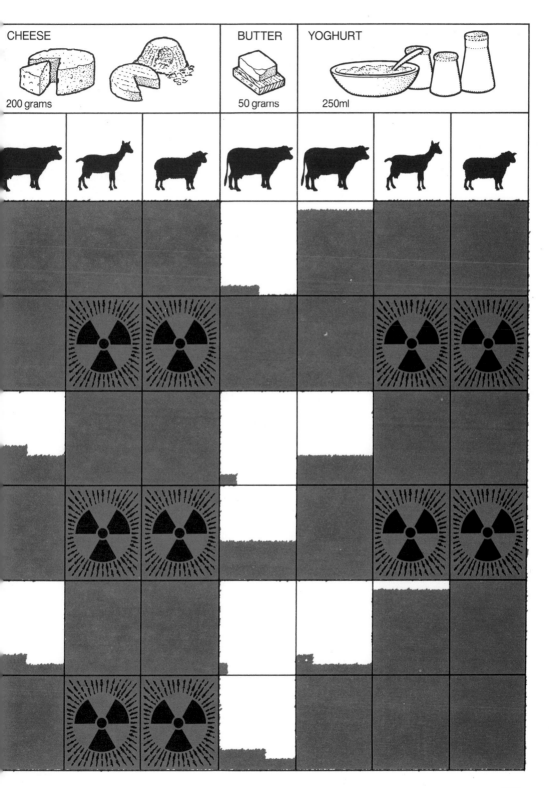

CHEESE			BUTTER	YOGHURT		
200 grams			50 grams	250ml		

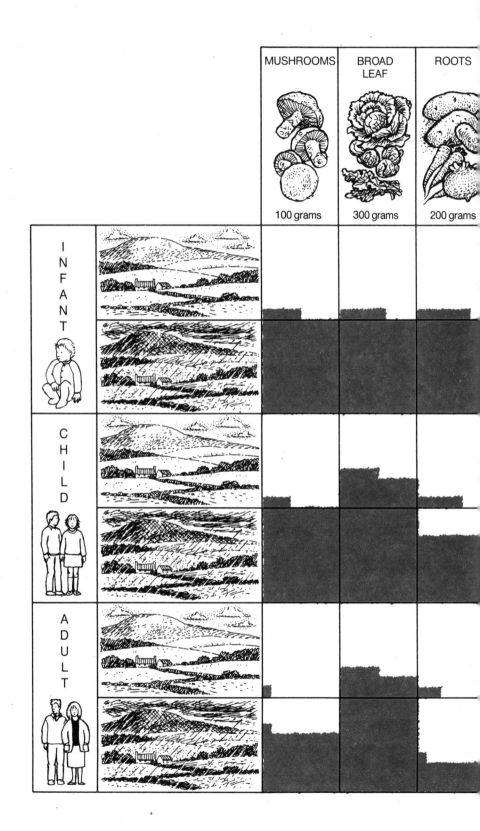

			MUSHROOMS	BROAD LEAF	ROOTS
			100 grams	300 grams	200 grams
INFANT					
CHILD					
ADULT					

GRAINS	HERBS	NUTS	SOFT FRUIT	APPLES & PEARS	STONED FRUIT	HONEY
300 grams	10 grams	50 grams	100 grams	100 grams	100 grams	100 grams
✓	✓	✓		✓		✓
✓	✓	✓	✓	✓		✓
✓	✓	✓	✓	✓		✓

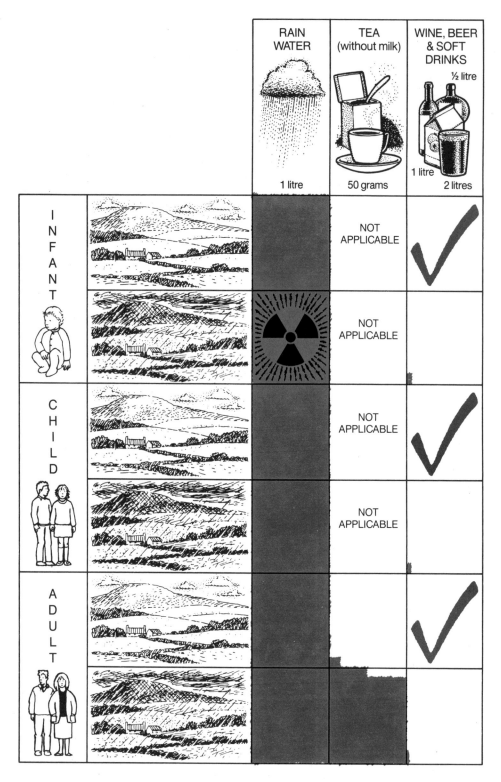

		RAIN WATER	TEA (without milk)	WINE, BEER & SOFT DRINKS
		1 litre	50 grams	½ litre / 1 litre / 2 litres
INFANT			NOT APPLICABLE	✓
			NOT APPLICABLE	
CHILD			NOT APPLICABLE	✓
			NOT APPLICABLE	
ADULT				✓

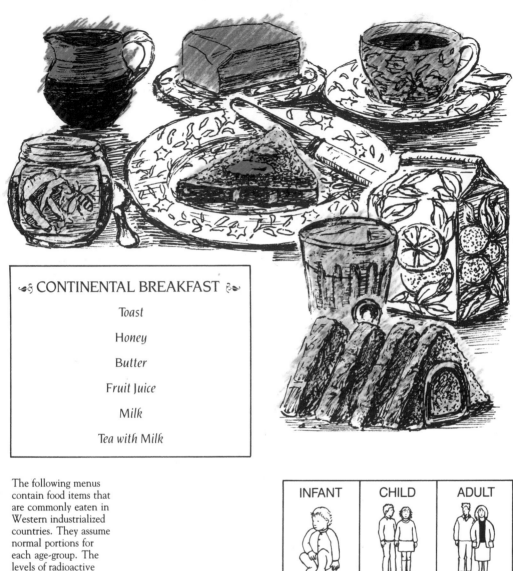

⊷§ CONTINENTAL BREAKFAST §⊷

Toast

Honey

Butter

Fruit Juice

Milk

Tea with Milk

The following menus contain food items that are commonly eaten in Western industrialized countries. They assume normal portions for each age-group. The levels of radioactive contamination for the foods are indicated by the intensity of red colour and are equivalent to the total contamination when a complete meal is eaten. It is assumed that a person continues to eat the same menu for a year, irrespective of any restrictions or bans. By studying these menus, it is possible to compile others and estimate their total radiation dose.

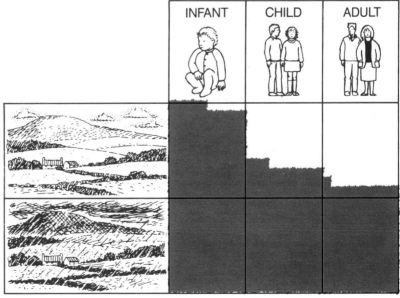

	INFANT	CHILD	ADULT

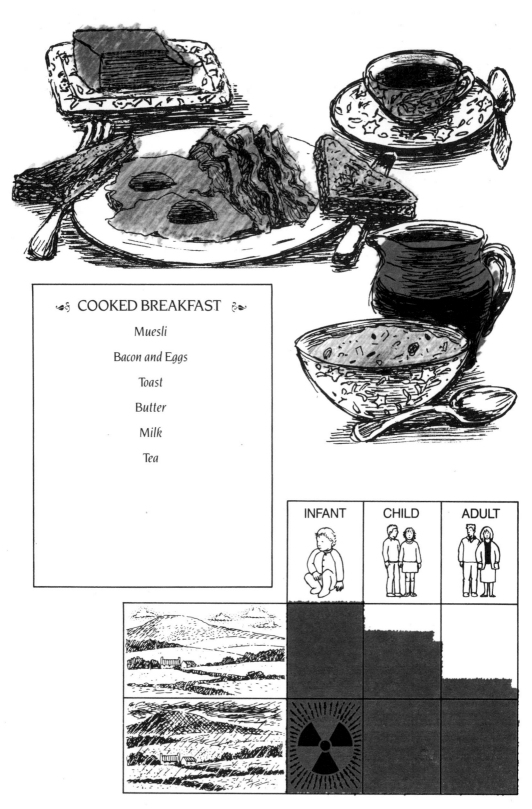

❧ COOKED BREAKFAST ❧

Muesli

Bacon and Eggs

Toast

Butter

Milk

Tea

	INFANT	CHILD	ADULT

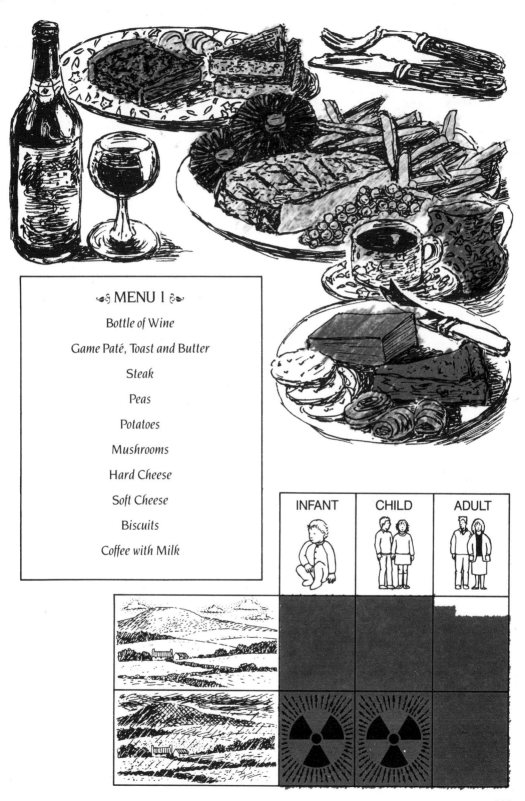

❧ MENU 1 ❧

Bottle of Wine

Game Paté, Toast and Butter

Steak

Peas

Potatoes

Mushrooms

Hard Cheese

Soft Cheese

Biscuits

Coffee with Milk

	INFANT	CHILD	ADULT

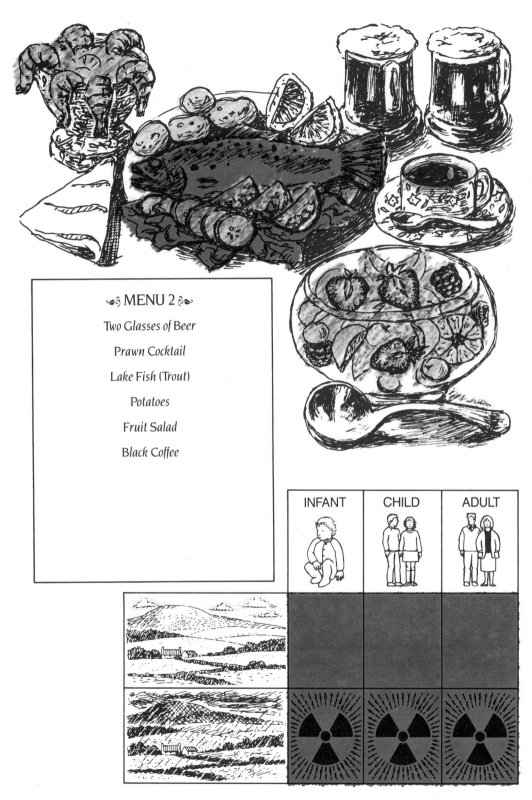

❧ MENU 2 ❧

Two Glasses of Beer

Prawn Cocktail

Lake Fish (Trout)

Potatoes

Fruit Salad

Black Coffee

INFANT	CHILD	ADULT

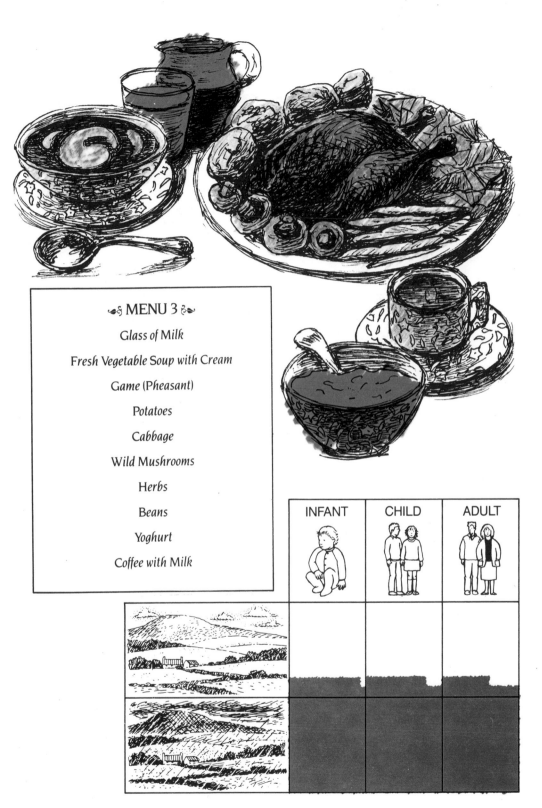

MENU 3

Glass of Milk

Fresh Vegetable Soup with Cream

Game (Pheasant)

Potatoes

Cabbage

Wild Mushrooms

Herbs

Beans

Yoghurt

Coffee with Milk

	INFANT	CHILD	ADULT

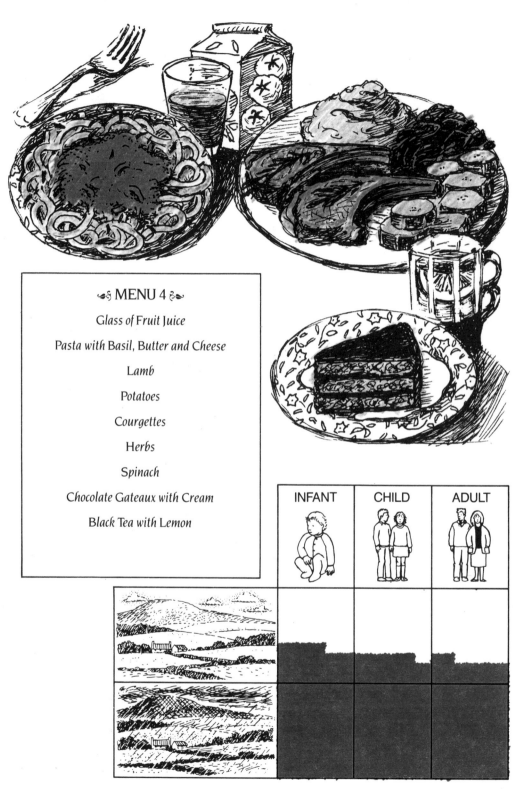

❧ MENU 4 ❧

Glass of Fruit Juice

Pasta with Basil, Butter and Cheese

Lamb

Potatoes

Courgettes

Herbs

Spinach

Chocolate Gateaux with Cream

Black Tea with Lemon

INFANT	CHILD	ADULT

APPENDIX

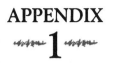

Notes on compiling the tables and charts for Chapter 6.

Milk

1. Iodine deposition on the ground dry:wet is taken as 1:15; caesium deposition is 5 times less than iodine in dry deposition and equivalent to it in wet deposition; strontium is taken as 2 per cent of caesium deposition under both dry and wet conditions.
2. For pasture, the interception factor from ground into grass is 0.25 for all three isotopes. Cows under usual conditions consume grass from 100 square metres a day, or its equivalent in hay (some 15 kilograms). The NRPB assumes 10 square metres of pasture are equivalent to one kilogram of dry grass.
3. For cows, the quantity of the isotopes consumed that goes into the milk are one per cent per litre for iodine and caesium, and 0.5 per cent for strontium. These results are taken from American data; however Sweden uses a transfer factor of 0.33 per cent per litre for caesium, and following Chernobyl the University of Constance Physics Department found 0.4 per cent.
4. For goats, the transfer factors are somewhat different according to American data. Thus 5 per cent per litre of the daily intake of iodine goes into the milk, and at least 10 per cent per litre of caesium. The factor for strontium is 1.4 per cent per litre. Meanwhile for sheep, according to one American authority, at least 10 per cent of the iodine consumed daily goes into the milk and 4 per cent of the strontium. The tables use a transfer factor of 10 per cent for caesium.
5. An effective decay constant to account for radioactive decay and weathering of 0.13 per day is used for iodine-131, and 0.05 per day for caesium-137, caesium-134 and strontium-90. Using these figures, the long-term doses to humans from a daily consumption of products without radiological restriction can be calculated. An original iodine deposition of 1,000 becquerels per square metre in grass gives a total whole-body effective dose to infants (one year old) of 0.8 millisieverts, assuming that a litre of cow's milk is drunk daily. An original deposition of 100 becquerels per square metre of caesium-137 gives the infant an effective whole-body dose of 0.15 millisievert when a litre of cow's milk is consumed daily.
6. The dose relationship between strontium and caesium is 1.74:1, taking into account the fact that strontium remains in the body much longer than caesium but only one-third of the strontium ingested gets taken into the body (whereas all the caesium is assumed to be absorbed).
7. For cheeses, the following factors are used compared to the radio-isotope content of milk: for iodine, a factor of 3; for caesium, a factor of 3 for soft cheeses and 1.5 for hard cheeses; for strontium, 7 for soft cheeses and 0.35 for hard cheeses. For butter the factors compared with milk are 0.4 for iodine, 0.1 for caesium and 0.07 for strontium. For cream, the factor from whole milk is 0.1 for iodine, 0.025 for caesium and 0 for strontium. Yoghurt is considered to be the same as whole milk.

Eggs, meat and fish

1. The ground deposition after Chernobyl was some 80,000 becquerels per square metre of iodine-131 and approximately 20,000 becquerels per square metre for caesium in the Lake Constance area of West Germany. This deposition on the ground led to the following results: For eggs, 560 becquerels per kilogram (approximately 20 becquerels per egg) for caesium. In the Constance region the average caesium levels in beef went up to 100 becquerels per kilogram, and in deer meat at least 600 becquerels. Meanwhile woodland deer grazing on the different soil conditions around Regensberg in Bavaria were discovered to have at least 30 times the quantities of caesium for just three times the caesium deposited at Constance, a factor difference of 10.
2. Iodine-131 consumption is unlikely to be significant in the dose if meat from contaminated areas is not consumed for at least one month after deposition has occurred.
3. In Cumbria, according to the British Ministry of Agriculture, some 30,000 becquerels per square

metre deposition of caesium led to levels of 1,000 becquerels and more per kilogram in lamb meat. In Constance, a deposition of 80,000 becquerels per square metre of iodine-131 led to game meat levels of up to 1,000 becquerels for iodine (and up to 300,000 becquerels per kilogram in the thyroid of deer). The tables assume similar iodine levels in sheep, namely 1,000 becquerels per kilogram for a deposition of 80,000 becquerels per square metre.

4. On 3 May 1986, following Chernobyl, the concentration in surface waters in Cumbria was some 12 becquerels per litre for iodine and 10 becquerels per litre for caesium. In 1982 the Irish Sea off Seascale had 10 becquerels per litre, indicating a rapid dispersal of the large quantities of caesium discharged from Sellafield into the sea. If the ground deposition of caesium after Chernobyl is taken as 30,000 becquerels per square metre in Cumbria, and that amount of deposition is assumed to have given rise to a level of contamination such as has actually been found in plaice and cod caught off Seascale in 1982, then the contamination is 400 becquerels per kilogram in cod and plaice, 300 becquerels per kilogram in lobsters, and 100 becquerels per kilogram in mussels.

5. In Swabia in West Germany, 5,000 becquerels per kilogram of caesium were found in fish in small lakes. Caesium tends to remain in the biogenic zones, at least during the summer.

Vegetables, cereals and fruits

1. Mushrooms retain absorbed radionuclides, thus the effective half-lives of long-lived isotopes such as caesium-137 is several years. Nevertheless a shorter effective half-life has been assumed. To convert dry weight into wet weight a factor of 10 has been used. In contaminated areas of France, mushrooms have been found with 15,000 becquerels per kilogram (dry weight).

2. NRPB data for Britain indicates that a deposition of iodine-131 of approximately 1,000 becquerels per square metre gave rise to a contamination of some 200 becquerels per kilogram by 6 May, and therefore to some 500 bec-

querels per kilogram at the beginning of May. At Constance in West Germany, spinach with 4,500 becquerels per kilogram was found on 14 May, equivalent to 36,000 becquerels per kilogram of iodine initially.

The NRPB found that for caesium a deposition of 100 becquerels per square metre gives a contamination in cabbage, spinach, and so on of 10 becquerels per kilogram.

3. Radishes and similar root crops were found to retain 6.5 becquerels of each 100 becquerels of iodine deposited, and 7.5 becquerels per 10,000 becquerels of caesium (at Constance).

Rye and barley are more contaminated for a particular level of fall-out than are wheat and oats. Thus the former have 10 times more caesium at approximately 5 becquerels per 1,000 becquerels of deposition. Cri du Rad data indicated that Mediterranean herbs have contamination levels of some 150 becquerels per kilogram for 1,000 becquerels of caesium deposited per square metre. Nuts were found to have 15 becquerels per 1,000 becquerels of fall-out; soft fruit 5 becquerels per 1,000 (iodine was 300 becquerels per 1,000 deposited). Stoned fruit such as cherries had 20 becquerels per 1,000 of caesium, apples and pears had 1.5 per 1,000, and honey 10 becquerels per 1,000.

Liquids

1. In Cumbria on 6 May 300 becquerels of iodine-131 were found per litre of rainwater – i.e., 600 becquerels on deposition. At the same time the caesium levels were 200 becquerels per litre. The tables assume that deposition in Cumbria was approximately 30,000 becquerels per square metre of both iodine and caesium.

2. According to investigation by AGöF in Bremen, Turkish black tea had up to 34,000 becquerels per kilogram of caesium and 100 becquerels of strontium.

3. Rainwater in Munich had 40 becquerels of caesium per litre and 0.4 per litre of strontium.

4. Wines from West Germany and Italy indicated levels of caesium of approximately 5 becquerels per litre. Apple juices had up to 15 becquerels per litre.

APPENDIX

2

Some data on radioactive contamination in Western Europe
following Chernobyl (figures in becquerels per kg or per litre)

Item	Place	Date	Caesium
Soil			
Garden soil	Saxony	Oct 86	892
Garden soil	W. Germany	Jan 87	1,228
Garden soil	W. Germany	May 87	1,870
Garden soil	W. Germany	June 87	2,257
Garden soil	France – Haut Rhine	July 87	458
Environment			
Air filter	W. Germany – Munich	Jan 87	84,120
Air filter	W. Germany – Munich	May 87	62,202
House dust	W. Germany	Oct 86	10,980
House dust	France	July 87	3,942
Lake water	France – Drome	May 86	6,228
Pine	W. Germany	Jan 87	17,340
Puddle water	UK – Highlands	May 86	1,100
Rain from gutter	W. Germany		736
River sand	W. Germany	June 87	165
River silt	W. Germany – Danube	Jan 87	12,222
Wood	W. Germany	Jan 87	33,504
Wood ash	W. Germany	June 87	11,476
Herbs and nuts			
Almonds	France	Oct 86	199
Bay leaves	W. Germany	May 87	198
Black tea	Turkey	Jan 87	40,350
Hazelnuts	Turkey	Aug 87	797
Hazelnuts	Italy	June 87	339
Hazelnuts	Corsica	June 86	337
Hazelnut spread	Saxony	June 87	475
Laurel	France	June 87	698
Nougat	W. Germany	June 87	124
Oregano	Turkey	Aug 87	1,033
Rosemary	France	June 87	927
Serpolet	France – Drome	June 87	2,357
Tea	Turkey	Oct 86	35,600
Tea	Georgia, Soviet Union	Jan 87	5,410
Thyme	France – Vaucluse	May 86	7,317
Thyme	France – Vaucluse	May 87	300
Thyme	France – Hautes Alpes	May 86	10,882

Item	Place	Date	Caesium
Fruits and vegetables			
Apples	Turkey	June 87	198
Bilberries	W. Germany		433
Blackcurrants	W. Germany	May 87	324
Bread	W. Germany – Bavaria	Nov 87	454
Broccoli	UK – Bedford	May 86	10
Cabbage	UK – Bedford	May 86	92
Cassis	France – Doubs	June 86	143
Cherries	W. Germany	May 87	179
Chestnuts	W. Germany	Nov 87	2,410
Leeks	UK – Bedford	May 86	115
Noodles	W. Germany		73
Spaghetti	Italy	Nov 87	77
Wheat	Greece	Aug 87	1,069
Milk and dairy products			
Baby food	W. Germany	Jan 87	183
Buttermilk	W. Germany	Jan 87	25
Chocolate (full milk)	W. Germany	Nov 87	159
Condensed milk	W. Germany	Jan 88	52
Condensed milk	UK – Scotland	May 86	588
Dry goat's cheese	France – Vaucluse	June 87	557
Ewe's milk	UK – Highlands	May 86	814
Fat-free milk	W. Germany	Jan 87	284
Goat's milk	France – Drome	March 87	125
Goat's milk	UK – Cumbria	May 86	351
Goat's cheese	France – Isere	Sep 86	327
Goat's cheese	France – Drome	May 86	4,396
Ice cream	W. Germany	June 87	30
Milk powder	W. Germany	Jan 87	5,806
Milk – rennet	France – Haut Rhine	May 87	106
Mother's milk	W. Germany	Jan 87	7
Mother's milk	France – Ardeche	June 87	17
Yoghurt	W. Germany	May 87	37
Meat			
Beef	W. Germany	May 87	404
Elk	W. Germany	Jan 87	259
Fawn	W. Germany	1987	362
Goat	France – Lozere	June 87	485
Lamb	France – Drome	April 87	1,054
Lamb	UK – Cumbria	May 86	2,450
Lamb's liver	UK – Cumbria	May 86	1,940
Mutton	W. Germany	May 87	1,004
Pork	W. Germany	Jan 87	102
Rabbit (farm)	France – Haut Rhine	Jan 87	464
Venison	W. Germany	1987	650
Venison	W. Germany	Jan 87	1,657
Wild boar	W. Germany	1987	716
Wool	W. Germany	1987	372
Wool	W. Germany	June 87	710
Wool	W. Germany	Nov 87	1,323

Item	Place	Date	Caesium
Fungi and honey			
Birch fungi	W. Germany	Oct 86	1,383
Cepes	France – Loire	Oct 86	7,399
Chanterelles	France – Loire	Nov 86	9,115
Edible fungi	W. Germany	1987	1,055
Edible fungi	W. Germany	Jan 87	2,020
Honey	Austria	May 87	171
Honey	W. Germany	Jan 88	84
Honey (spruce)	France – Vaucluse	1986	234
Lichens	Corsica	May 87	8,454
Lichens	France – Alpes Maritimes	Apr 87	3,755
Moss	W. Germany	Jan 88	26,638
Moss	Corsica	May 87	5,276
Mushrooms	W. Germany	Nov 87	14,289
Pollen	France – Var	Oct 86	229
Wild edible fungi	East Germany	1987	6,691
Grass and hay			
Compost	W. Germany	Oct 86	132
Grass	W. Germany	May 87	295
Grass deposition	UK Cumbria	May 86	26,307
Hay	W. Germany	Jan 87	6,860
Hay	Corsica	June 86	2,450
Hay	W. Germany	May 87	15,382
Hay	France – Drome	June 86	10,491
Hay – 1st cut	France – Haut Rhin	July 86	1,696
Hay silage	W. Germany	Jan 87	3,610
Manure	W. Germany	Nov 87	482

Some samples taken from the Soviet Union and Eastern Europe soon after the Chernobyl Accident and measured by the NRPB in Britain

Item	Place	Date	Caesium	Iodine-131
Cherries (immature)	Bucharest	8 May 86	14,000	32,000
Grapes (immature)	Bucharest	7 May 86	20,000	38,000
Grass	Bucharest	3 May 86	8,000	20,000
Grass	Warsaw	4 May 86	2,590	7,000
Grass (deposition)	Moscow	3 May 86	1,000	3,200
Leaf (4ft above ground)	Kiev	5 May 86	69,000	1.3 million
Lettuce	Bucharest	4 May 86	850	3,200
Lettuce	Bucharest	7 May 86	3,700	12,000
Lettuce	Warsaw	5 May 86	170	3,000
Milk	Warsaw	5 May 86	40	210
Milk	Warsaw	9 May 86	53	430
Parsley	Bucharest	4 May 86	660	2,600
Radish	Bucharest	8 May 86	2,000	3,500
Spinach	Bucharest	7 May 86	850	4,000
Spinach (unwashed)	Moscow	7 May 86	13	470

The sources for the above information were:

Arbeitsgemeinschaft ökologischer Forschungsinstitute (AGöF)
Commission Regionale Indépendante d' Information sur la Radioactivè (CRII-RAD)
UK National Radiological Protection Board (NRPB)

APPENDIX

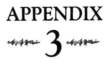

3

In 1987 the European Economic Community agreed the following
radiation limits (expressed in becquerels per kg), to come
into force on 1 November 1987.

Radio-isotope	Dairy produce*	Other foods	Drinking water	Animal feed
Strontium-90 and iodine-131	500	3,000	400	–
Plutonium-239 and americium-241	20	80	10	–
Caesium-134 and caesium-137	1,000	1,250	800	2,500

* including baby food

APPENDIX 4

Radiation risk

New studies on the radiation dose received by survivors of the Hiroshima and Nagasaki atomic bombs have forced the International Authority (ICRP) to reassess dramatically its cancer-risk estimates. The previous projection was one extra cancer death for every 100 sieverts of radiation. It is now thought that the real figure might be twice this number, and perhaps even higher. Indeed, some scientists claim that the risk of radiation causing cancer may be 15 times higher than the one extra cancer death per 100 sieverts.

Despite accepting the new data and the resulting conclusions, the ICRP decided in September 1987 to keep the recommended permissible levels for the general population as they stand – 1 millisievert per year from radiation other than natural background and medical sources.

The National Radiological Protection Board of Britain, however, believes that action must be taken now. In an unprecedented move the NRPB has broken ranks with the ICRP, stating that the new estimates of risk would make the previous permissible levels unacceptably high.

The NRPB now bases its recommendations on a risk of one extra cancer death in 1,000 each year being acceptable for workers in the nuclear industry, and one in 100,000 each year being acceptable for the general population. Therefore, taking the risk as 3 extra cancer deaths for every 100 sieverts exposure, a worker exposed close to the 50 millisievert limit over his working life would increase the risk of dying of cancer by some 6 per cent. This increase is in addition to the normal risk, which for males works out at 20 per cent on average. For the worker, therefore, the present ICRP limit would give a risk in excess of one in 1,000. The NRPB has therefore recommended that the limit for people exposed occupationally to radiation should be reduced by at least three-fold to 15 millisieverts in a year.

For the general population, particularly in view that some members of the public are exposed to higher levels of natural background radiation than others, depending on where they live, the NRPB recommends that the maximum exposure to any one individual from a nuclear installation should not exceed 0.5 millisieverts in a year.

At present some 800 workers, or 14 per cent of the workforce at a nuclear installation such as the reprocessing plant at Sellafield in Cumbria, receive yearly doses in excess of the 15-millisievert recommended limit. Equally some members of the public in the vicinity of Sellafield have received doses during a year in excess of 0.5 millisieverts.

At the same time, should the radiation risk prove to be 15 or even 20 times greater than that underlying the current ICRP dose limits, then the NRPB's recommendations will themselves need to be reduced by at least another five times. Whether the nuclear industry could operate such stringent limits is a moot point.

GLOSSARY

actinides Elements such as plutonium, neptunium and americium, all of which have atomic numbers higher than 89.

activation product Previously stable atoms that become radioactive through intense neutron bombardment in certain materials used in the structure of a nuclear reactor. Nickel and niobium in steel, for instance, can absorb neutrons and become strong gamma-emitters, thus creating difficulties during dismantling of the reactor and disposal of the pieces.

alpha-emmiter Radioactive substance, such as plutonium, that in decaying discharges an alpha particle.

alpha particle Package of two neutrons and two protons bound together which, because of a relatively large mass, has considerable energy on leaving the nucleus of the original atom. An alpha particle has a net positive charge of two units, and can cause intense localized damage in body tissues.

atom Smallest particle of an element that preserves its identity, consisting of various subparticles, the most important of which are neutrons, protons and orbiting electrons.

atomic mass Mass of an atom, equal to the total masses of all its protons and neutrons.

atomic number Number of protons in an atom, equal also to the number of electrons in the unionized atom. The number of protons determine which element it is. Hydrogen, for instance, has one proton, helium two, and carbon six protons.

atomic weight Old term for *atomic mass*.

background radiation Natural radiation derived from cosmic and terrestrial sources. The actual amount varies with location: at high altitudes there is more cosmic radiation than at sea level, and some regions of the Earth have high terrestrial radiation from deposits of uranium and thorium. On average every person receives some 2 millisieverts of background radiation each year.

becquerel Unit of radioactivity equal to one atomic disintegration per second.

beta particle Equivalent to an electron, discharged from a nucleus. It comes from a neutron, and because it is itself negatively charged, leaves the neutron with a positive charge so that it transforms into a proton. Thus, when a beta particle is emitted from an atom, the *atomic number* goes up by one although the *atomic mass* remains very nearly the same. Like alpha particles, beta particles cause ionizing radiation.

burn-up Amount of energy that can be derived from nuclear fuel before it is considered spent. It is usually measured in terms of megawatt-days per tonne of fuel. The higher the enrichment of the fuel with fissile material (such as uranium-235 or plutonium), the higher the burn-up that can be achieved. Fast reactors with fuel enriched to 15 per cent or more can achieve fuel burn-ups in the range of 100,000 megawatt-days per tonne, compared to some 5,000 megawatt-days per tonne for a reactor such as a Magnox using natural unenriched uranium with a fissile content of only 0.7 per cent.

chain reaction Sequence of events that occur when one fissioning atom releases enough neutrons to bring about the fissioning of another atom, and so on, in a continuous chain. When this occurs in a reactor it is considered to have achieved criticality. Control of a chain reaction at a particular constant level is achieved through adjustments of the *control rods*.

containment Reinforced concrete or steel structure that encloses a reactor, designed to withstand minor explosions in the core and to keep in escaping radionuclides.

contamination Any incident in which buildings, land or people become contaminated with radioactive waste (as during accidents).

control rod Part of a nuclear reactor that includes such neutron-absorbers as steel, boron and cadmium, which moves between the reactor fuel, adjusting the reactor power, and if necessary shutting off the chain reaction.

core Part of the reactor that contains the fuel and coolant.

cosmic radiation Radiation from outer space, much of which is stopped by the upper layers of the atmosphere. Some cosmic radiation is extremely energetic and able to penetrate a mile or more into the Earth.

critical group In a particular environment, following radioactive fall-out, certain groups of people (children or families with a particular lifestyle) who may be more likely to expose themselves to radiation compared with other people. The authorities assume that if a careful watch is kept on the most exposed group – the critical group – to see that nobody in that group receives more than the maximum permissible level, then other members of the population will be at a lower risk.

curie Number of disintegrations per second emanating from one gram of radium; it is equivalent to 3.7×10^{10} (37 thousand million) disintegrations per second.

decommission To dismantle a nuclear installation. The notion is to make the site safe, either by taking away and disposing of the pieces or by covering the site with a protective layer so as to keep down radiation doses to the public.

dumping Disposal of nuclear waste. Where to put radioactive waste has become a major public issue and the authorities have increasingly to deal with the 'Not in my backyard' syndrome. Proposed schemes vary from sending radioactive waste out into space to dumping it so that it gets taken deep into the Earth.

effective dose Radiation dose to a specific organ in the body can be estimated in terms of a dose to the whole body by using a weighting factor specific to the organ in question. For instance, a dose of 1 sievert to the thyroid translates into a whole-body dose by multiplying it by the weighting factor for the thyroid of 0.03. The whole-body dose estimated in such a way is known as an effective dose.

electron Negatively-charged sub-atomic particle of much smaller mass than a proton. A neutral atom is in a balanced electrical state, when the number of electrons orbiting the nucleus is equal to the number of protons.

element Atom with a distinct number of protons, thus conferring on it a specific chemical identity.

fall-out Radioactive substances carried in the wind and gradually deposited on the ground. Rain falling through a radioactive plume washes out volatile particles at an accelerated rate.

fast reactor Nuclear reactor that has no *moderator* to slow down the neutrons used to bring about the chain reaction. The idea of such reactors is to generate more plutonium than they burn by surrounding the core with a blanket of uranium-238.

Fast reactors use liquid metallic sodium to take heat out of the core.

fissile Able to undergo nuclear fission; generally applied to uranium-235, plutonium-239 or uranium-233.

fission Splitting of an atom with the release of energy. For instance, a neutron striking a uranium or plutonium atom may cause it to split into two more-or-less equal halves, with the release of more neutrons and energy.

free radicals Very reactive species of an atom or group of atoms. Ionizing radiation can strip electrons from atoms and leave them in an ionized state. Water, for instance, can be split by such ionizing into a highly reactive oxidizing compound called hydroxyl. Such substances combine swiftly and powerfully with other chemical compounds in their immediate vicinity. Free radicals are therefore agents of chemical transformation and derangement.

gamma rays High-energy photons with considerable penetrating power, needing a slab of lead or concrete to stop them. Gamma rays are emitted during the radioactive decay of certain elements, and can cause ionizations as they pass through matter.

gigawatt Measure of power equal to 1,000 million watts (10^9 watts). The latest nuclear reactors being built are in the one-gigawatt range.

graphite Natural form of carbon. It acts as a good *moderator* in a nuclear reactor, slowing down fast neutrons to slow thermal speed after some hundred collisions. It does not appreciably absorb neutrons in slowing them down.

gray Radiation unit equal to one joule per kilogram, and therefore 100 times larger than a rad. When multiplied by a biological quality factor to account for the difference between the effects on tissues of the various radiation types (such as alpha particles, beta radiation and gamma-rays), the gray converts into the *sievert* and the rad into the *rem*.

half-life Period of time taken by half the number of atoms of a radioactive substance to decay. Over each successive half-life, half of the atoms remaining undergo decay, so that after two half-lives one quarter of the original amount is left, and after three half-lives just one-eighth.

ion Atom or group of atoms carrying an electrical charge. The loss of an electron from an atom produces a positively-charged ion (thus removing an electron from a hydrogen atom gives a hydrogen ion H^+). Many non-metallic elements form negative ions (such as chloride, Cl^-).

ionizing radiation Radiation that causes electrons to be stripped away from an atom (to form ions). Such radiation therefore causes fundamental changes in the chemistry of substance in the cells in the body, and can bring about the death of a cell or its transformation into a malignant one.

inert gas Gas such as neon, argon, xenon and krypton that does not readily undergo chemical reactions. Some, such as argon, xenon and krypton, can be made radioactive in a reactor through fission processes.

isotope Species of a chemical element with a different *atomic mass* (but the same *atomic number*). The chemical nature of a particular element is a property of the number of protons in the nucleus (atomic number) although in some elements the number of neutrons may vary, and the atomic mass changes accordingly. Atoms of an element with differing neutron numbers are known as isotopes. Uranium-235, for instance, has 92 protons and 146 neutrons, whereas the uranium-235 isotope has 92 protons and only 143 neutrons. Some isotopes are stable (carbon-12, for example); others (carbon-14, for example) are unstable.

latency Time taken after an initiating event for a cancer to manifest itself.

meltdown Melting of the fuel in a nuclear reactor caused by loss of coolant. The danger is that the molten fuel may burn its way through the reactor pressure vessel and containment, as well as giving rise to inflammable gases such as hydrogen.

micro- One millionth, often used in association with sieverts.

milli- One-thousandth, hence millirem or millisievert. Average background radiation, for instance, is approximately 200 millirems per year, or 2,000 microsievert.

moderator Substance that, in a nuclear reactor, slows down neutrons to thermal speeds through a series of collisions. Moderators have to be composed of light elements such as hydrogen, deuterium or carbon. Thus light water, heavy water or graphite are used, depending on the reactor type.

molecule Combination of atoms to form a composite with physical and chemical properties different from that of the individual components. Molecules vary in size from the combination of two hydrogen atoms (to form hydrogen gas) to polymers and the macro protein molecules found in a living cell.

neutrons Particle of similar mass to a proton, but without any electrical charge. Neutrons are released from uranium and plutonium during fissioning, and by colliding with other fissile atoms can cause more fissioning, thereby bringing about a *chain reaction*.

non-ionizing radiation Radiation such as thermal radiation (heat) and light – even ultraviolet light which, although it can damage cells and tissues, does not involve ionizing events.

nuclear waste Unwanted by-products of controlled nuclear reactions. The fissioning of uranium or plutonium gives rise to a host of fission products which are highly radioactive, and must be kept isolated from the environment into the distant future. The spent reactor fuel contains unused uranium and plutonium as well as nuclear waste, and *reprocessing* is used to separate one from the other.

nucleus Central part of an atom that contains the protons and neutrons. In a living cell, the nucleus consists of the genetic material (deoxyribonucleic acid, or DNA) bound by a special membrane.

overburden Top layers of soil and rock that have to be shifted to expose a mineral ore.

person-sievert When a group of people are subjected to a blanket dose of radiation, as for instance following the discharge of radioactive waste from a nuclear installation, the total dose can be evaluated in terms of sieverts multiplied by the number of people involved. Thus one millisievert received by 1,000 people gives a total dose of one person-sievert.

photons Packets of energy that comprise all electromagnetic radiation, such as light, radio waves, gamma-rays and X-rays. At low energies they are non-ionizing; at higher energies they are ionizing. Photons can be thought of as minute particles without any mass that travel at the speed of light.

plume Gases and volatile particles expelled into the atmosphere after a nuclear accident. Although gradually dispersing, the plume remains relatively intact even after several thousand kilometres of being carried by the wind.

prompt/delayed neutrons Prompt neutrons are released during the fissioning of fissile material; delayed neutrons are released later, sometimes seconds after the radioactive decay of fission products. A reactor achieves criticality when the *chain reaction* is sustained by the contribution of both kinds of neutrons.

PWR Abbreviation of pressurized water reactor,

so-named because the water in the pressure vessel is under such high pressure – approximately 170 atmospheres – that it does not boil. The water acts simultaneously as moderator and coolant.

rad Radiation dose in terms of its energy. One rad is 100 ergs per gram, or 0.01 joules per kilogram.

radioactive decay In-built tendency of radioactive substances to shed atomic particles and transform into different elements.

radioactivity Result of sudden, unpredictable transformations of atoms that are inherently unstable into atoms of an entirely different element. Such events are marked by the expulsion of particles (such as *alpha* or *beta particles*) and the release of energy in the form of heat and *gamma-rays*. Occasionally certain atoms merely expel a neutron, and they therefore remain the same element but with a smaller mass.

radio-iodine Radioactive *isotope* of iodine.

radio-isotope Isotope of an element that is unstable and radioactive.

radionuclide Any element that is radioactive.

radon Alpha-emitting radioactive gas that is a decay product of radium. Radon tends to seep out of the ground and accumulate in building basements. It has a short half-life of a few days, but its own decay products are also intensely radioactive. High levels of radon are now implicated in causing lung cancer.

reactor Vessel, core, coolant and control systems of an atomic generator.

reactor scram Quick, emergency shut-down of a nuclear reactor brought about by dropping the *control rods* into the core.

refuelling Replacing spent fuel in a nuclear reactor. Most reactors need to be shut down to be refuelled, the spent fuel rods being pulled out of the core by remote control and replaced by fresh ones. Some reactor types, such as CANDU or Magnox, can be refuelled while still operating.

rem Acronym for röntgen-equivalent-man, an older term now being replaced by sievert. One rem is equivalent to one-hundredth of a sievert.

reprocessing Chemical process by which plutonium and uranium in spent fuel are separated from the remaining fission products. Reprocessing gives rise to large volumes of *radioactive waste*, some of it (intensely radioactive) kept in specially cooled stainless steel tanks

until such time as it can be solidified and disposed of.

sievert Radiation dose to tissues, adjusted for the kind of radiation involved. For instance, alpha radiation is estimated to have 10 to 20 times greater impact dose for dose on the tissues of the body compared with gamma radiation or X-rays. The sievert is equal to one joule of radiation energy per kilogram of tissue multiplied by the quality factor for the type of radiation.

spent fuel Reactor fuel that has been in a reactor and in which fission products have built up to the point at which they poison (or slow down or stop) the chain reaction.

steam generator Basically a boiler in which steam is raised to turn electricity generating turbines. In pressure water reactors (*PWRs*) the steam generators consist of many small-bore tubes containing water at high pressure from the reactor coolant circuit, passing through a volume of water at much lower pressure. When heat is transferred to the low-pressure circuit, steam is formed.

terawatt-hour Million million watts (10^{12} watts) over the period of an hour. A one-gigawatt reactor working for three-quarters of a year at full power generates some 6.6 terawatt-hours of electricity.

transuranic Any element that has an atomic number greater than 92 (that of uranium).

uranium Element with 92 protons in its nucleus and therefore one of the heaviest elements found naturally on Earth. Always radioactive, it comes in two main forms: as the heavier uranium-238 isotope and the much rarer uranium-235 isotope. Uranium-235 is the only natural substance able to undergo fission. On the other hand, uranium-238 may capture a neutron in a reactor and form plutonium which, like uranium-235, is fissile. A third route to obtaining fissile material is to bombard thorium-232 with neutrons as in a High Temperature Reactor so that fissile uranium-233 is formed.

X-rays Artificially created electromagnetic radiation, commonly used for medical and scientific purposes. They consist of high-energy photons similar to, but less powerful than, *gamma-rays*.

Index